Pregnancy After Thirty

Pregnancy After Thirty

MARY ANDERSON
MB, ChB, FRCOG

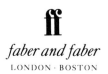

faber and faber
LONDON · BOSTON

First published in 1984
by Faber and Faber Limited
3 Queen Square London WC1N 3AU

Filmset by Wilmaset Birkenhead
Printed in Great Britain by
Redwood Burn Limited
Trowbridge Wiltshire
All rights reserved

© Mary Anderson 1984

British Library Cataloguing in Publication Data

Anderson, Mary
Pregnancy after thirty
1. Pregnancy   2. Childbirth
I. Title
618.2   RG524
ISBN 0–571–13355–X

To Susan, barrister,
whose idea it was to write this book

Contents

ILLUSTRATIONS

TABLES

Author's preface

It is a phenomenon of modern life that many women are establishing themselves in careers well into their late 20s or early 30s before contemplating marriage. After marriage they frequently want to continue working for a year or two before starting a family.

Some are worried about delaying their first pregnancy to this extent .and are anxious to be reassured, and given informed advice on any risks or problems which may arise.

A young friend of mine in just such a situation searched the bookstalls for information but failed to find it. With her encouragement I have attempted an appraisal of the facts for the older woman planning her first pregnancy. It is to be hoped that the result provides answers to most of her questions.

1

Age and reproduction

In almost every textbook of obstetrics (the science of midwifery) there is to be found a section with the title 'The Elderly Primigravida'. 'Primigravida' is the word used to describe a woman who is having her first baby. 'Elderly' is a word used by most people to describe someone who is old by any standards, an old age pensioner, a frail, white-haired being who is well into the latter period of life. In spite of this, the use of the word 'elderly' persists among obstetricians and it can do nothing for the morale of an older mother in her first pregnancy to hear herself described in this way. It strikes a definitely pessimistic note, so let us keep away from it in these pages and use the word 'older' instead.

Why is there any need to have special mention in textbooks of this group of women? Why are women uneasy about delaying their pregnancies sometimes until 30 or over? Are their fears justified and what can be done to reassure and help them? As is so often the case, newspapers, magazines and television have made women aware of problems and difficulties which they might never have known about otherwise. This is probably no bad thing since the subject is thereby aired, thought about and discussed, hopefully losing some of its fear in the process. But a little knowledge is indeed a potentially dangerous thing and a half-understanding of such a topic as the older mother and her pregnancy can only lead to considerable fears and tensions which may even cause further deferment of pregnancy.

It is to be hoped that this little book will answer a lot of such questions while not concealing facts and figures. At all times a mother should and must ask her attendant obstetrician to clarify any doubts she may have and to give her reassurance and explanation wherever possible. It must be stated quite categorically right at the beginning of our discussion that the majority of women having their first baby after the age of 30 will run a perfectly normal course throughout pregnancy, will give spontaneous birth to a normal healthy baby and will be well and happy afterwards.

Never forget this fact and do not get obsessed by lists of possible complications – they may never happen.

What is older?

It seems that the ideal age to have a baby is somewhere between 20 and 29, some would say 20 and 25. 'Reproductive performance' is a phrase used to cover many aspects of conception, pregnancy, labour, delivery and the postnatal period and it includes such things as delay in conceiving (over one year, for example), complications of pregnancy such as raised blood pressure, some bleeding problems, prolonged labour with a higher chance of instrumental or operative delivery, and so on. If we take women's 'reproductive performance' in relation to age we can indeed find a decline, certainly over the age of 40, in many aspects over the age of 35 and in some ways over the age of 25. So what are we to regard as older? If we take over the age of 25, we are strictly speaking quite correctly but obviously carrying the whole thing a bit too far. Thus many authorities would say over the age of 40, although mostly we take 35 years and over. The years between 30 and 35 are still in the older group and most obstetricians would want to keep a particularly close eye on such a mother even though she does not fit into the usually accepted statistical groups. To the majority of potential mothers, however, it does seem to be a source of anxiety not to have started a family by the late 20s and certainly by the early 30s. What are these worries; what are the questions that arise in their minds? I think that they lie in three main groups – with lots of subsidiary questions related to them.

1.   What can I do to ensure that I preserve my health and my childbearing ability so that when the time comes I will have no difficulty in conceiving, will remain healthy during my pregnancy and deliver a normal healthy baby?

2.   What are the possible risks to myself and to my baby if I defer having my first baby until I am over 30 or even over 35?

3.   If there are risks what can be done to minimise them and to safeguard myself and my baby?

These and their associated questions are what I hope to answer in this book. Let me remind you again, however, that the majority of older women will achieve their pregnancy easily, will pass through pregnancy normally and deliver their healthy babies safely. And remember, too, that the art and science of obstetrics has advanced rapidly over the past few years, and the obstetrician can nowadays use a variety of marvellous aids to watch over the older mother and her baby and so ensure a happy outcome for her and her partner.

2

The physiology of reproduction

It is not intended to discuss the functioning of woman's reproductive system in any great detail. For one thing, most interested and thoughtful women have learned about it long before marriage or even before having intercourse and, for another, there are many books which describe at length how a woman's body works. An outline scheme of things may not go amiss, however, as it is obviously relevant to much of what is discussed later. A fundamental knowledge of female anatomy is assumed.

Ovulation and menstruation

Each month – and the average monthly cycle is 28 days – a sequence of events occurs in the ovary gland aimed at producing an egg or ovum which is capable of being fertilised. These events can be summarised as follows (Fig. 1):

1.   A part of the brain called the hypothalamus produces chemical substances known as hormones which act on the front part of the pituitary gland (a tiny pea-sized structure lying at the base of the brain).

2.   The pituitary gland as a result produces two hormones called

      – follicle stimulating hormone (FSH) and

      – luteinising hormone (LH).

3.   The mature ovary is filled with follicles, which are tiny fluid-filled structures containing the egg cells. There are about 200 000 of these.

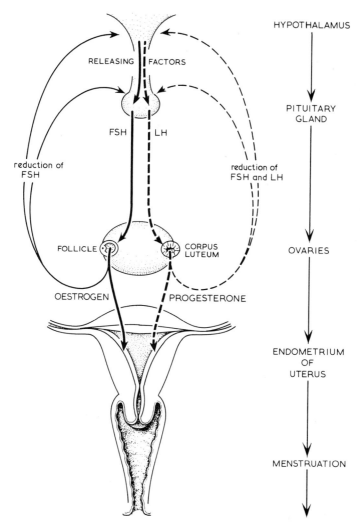

HYPOTHALAMUS

RELEASING FACTORS

PITUITARY
GLAND

FSH LH

reduction of
FSH

reduction of
FSH and LH

OVARIES

FOLLICLE

CORPUS
LUTEUM

OESTROGEN

PROGESTERONE

ENDOMETRIUM
OF
UTERUS

MENSTRUATION

Fig. 1 Control of menstruation

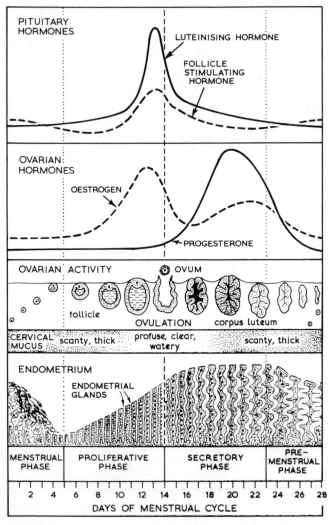

Fig. 2 Schematic description of menstruation and ovulation

One of these follicles comes to the surface of the ovary each month, stimulated by FSH, ruptures and sheds an ovum. Ovulation has taken place – an event actually initiated by a rise of LH.

4. During growth of the follicle the hormone oestrogen is produced. After the ovum has been shed the follicle collapses on itself to form a tiny yellowish-red structure called the corpus luteum and from this is produced the hormone progesterone.

5. Meantime, while these events are occurring in the ovary, the lining of the womb (the endometrium) has been influenced by the hormones oestrogen and progesterone. First it becomes thicker and develops more blood vessels. This is the effect of *oestrogen* and is known as the proliferative phase of the cycle. Next it becomes much thicker and 'juicier' with many blood vessels and glands filled with secretion. This is the effect of *progesterone*, known as the secretory phase, and the end result is to provide a rich nourishing bed for the ovum to settle down in should it be fertilised.

6. If fertilisation does not occur then the corpus luteum degenerates, the levels of oestrogen and progesterone fall so that the thick endometrium can no longer be sustained and it sloughs off, appearing as blood, called menstruation.

These events are difficult to remember even though their description has been simplified. Table 1 and Figure 2 summarise what happens, giving the time scale and a graphic record of both the ovarian and the endometrial cycle.

As a woman gets older two things happen. First, it is more common for the older woman to have what are known as anovular cycles. This means that although she menstruates, an ovum is not produced in mid-cycle. Ovulation is not essential for regular periods but not infrequently lack of ovulation is associated with irregular, often prolonged cycles. Quite obviously if ovulation only occurs occasionally that woman is

		No. of days
	Table 1. Summary of events leading to menstruation	
1.	After menstruation a follicle ripens: oestrogen is produced: the endometrium proliferates	10
2.	Ovulation	
3.	The corpus luteum appears: progesterone is produced: small amounts of oestrogen persist: the endometrium becomes secretory	14
4.	The corpus luteum degenerates: oestrogen and progesterone levels fall: menstruation	4
	TOTAL	28

going to find that it takes her longer to fall pregnant than the woman who ovulates regularly every month. Hence there may be a delay in conception for the older woman.

And another fact may influence the speed with which conception occurs. Over the years the eggs are gradually used up and it has been calculated that at the age of 40 only 5000 remain of the 200 000 present at puberty. Not only do the numbers diminish but the follicles may become less responsive to the influence of the pituitary hormones. But it must be stressed that both anovular cycles and significant reduction of egg cells are more commonly seen in much older age groups than we are considering here.

Conception

Conception occurs when a sperm penetrates the ovum. The sequence of events leading up to this is as follows:

The physiology of reproduction

1. The end of a healthy tube hanging over the ovary consists of finger-like processes which pick up the freed egg or ovum, which is then wafted down the tube by the hair-like processes on the surface of the tube's lining cells.

An egg has a life of about 24–36 hours.

2. Meanwhile, of the millions of sperms that are deposited in the semen at the time of intercourse and cover the upper vagina and cervix, some hundreds of thousands enter the cavity of the uterus but only thousands pass into the tubes.

A few hundred reach the outer portion of the tube where the ovum lies and a few penetrate the ovum's outer covering. Only one, however, gets to the very centre of the ovum fusing with the female nucleus – and then conception has occurred (Fig. 3a).

Sperms have a life of about 48 hours so it is worth noting perhaps that for fertilisation to occur, coitus must take place within two days of ovulation. Put another way, to achieve a pregnancy, coitus should take place every one to two days, around the time of ovulation.

3. When the ovum is fertilised it divides itself into a little ball of cells which is called a morula (Fig. 3b). The morula is wafted down the tube towards the cavity of the uterus and it reaches its destination about seven days after ovulation, that is about day 21 of the cycle. It settles into the thickened lining of the cavity and is fully embedded by the 14th day after ovulation, that is about day 28 of the cycle (Fig. 3c).

4. The endometrium, which you will remember was in the second half of its growth (the secretory phase) after ovulation, becomes even thicker and more 'lush' with plenty of blood supply. This is brought about by the continuing influence of the corpus luteum which, in turn, is directed by the pituitary hormones. This extra-thick vascular lining, obviously an ideal nest for the egg to settle into and be nourished by, now gets the name of the decidua.

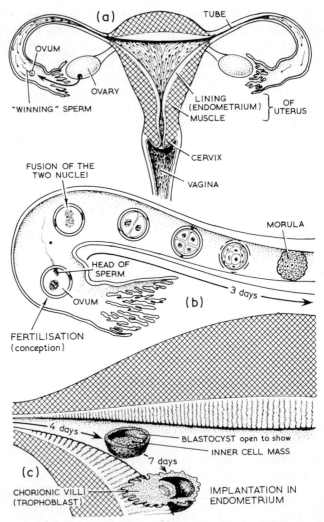

Fig. 3 Fertilisation. (a). The meeting of the sperm and ovum in the tube. (b). The developing cell. (c). Implantation into endometrium

5. To complete the picture, what has been happening meanwhile to the little ball of cells – the morula – the fertilised egg? By the time it has reached the end of its journey down the tube a small fluid-filled space has appeared to separate the morula into an outer shell with a mound of cells lying to one side. The outer shell of cells will become the placenta and the mound of cells, called the inner cell mass, will be the site of the development of the fetus.

The placenta takes over the production of the hormones required to maintain the corpus luteum which in its turn, you will remember, is producing hormones to sustain the growth of the decidua into which the fertilised egg is embedding. Later in pregnancy – after 10–12 weeks – the level of these hormones declines, the corpus luteum fails but the developing placenta takes over the production of oestrogen and progesterone.

Development and growth of the fetus

The story of the growth and development of the baby from the earliest group of cells, like a mulberry, to the fully formed mature baby after nine months or so is a fascinating one. Unfortunately it is not really relevant to the theme of this book, but for those who are interested it is well worth reading an account and studying some of the amazing photographs which are now available (see p. 120 for book titles). What may be of interest here, and of some relevance to the older mother worried about effects of drugs, for instance, on her developing baby, is to show you a time-table of events (Table 2). 'Differentiation' means the beginning of development of an organ or structure.

This then is an outline of the physiology of reproduction. The older woman is no different from the younger in any respect except that perhaps, as has been said, she may not

Table 2. Developmental times of the fetus – by weeks

	Differentiation	Complete formation
Spinal cord	3–4	20
Brain	3	28
Eyes	3	20–24
Ears (hearing apparatus)	3–4	24–28
Lungs	5	24–28
Heart	3	6
Intestinal system	3	24
Kidneys	3–4	12
Genital organs	5	7
Face	3–4	8
Limbs	4–5	8

ovulate quite so regularly. But once a pregnancy has been achieved its growth and development are the same in all ages. Of course one chief worry which older women have is whether their baby will grow and develop normally and this is something which we will consider in greater detail later.

3

Preparation for pregnancy

It seems that many of the anxieties of the older woman relate not so much to the problems that might arise when she does become pregnant but rather to the question of what she can do to maintain her fertility and how she can easily and quickly achieve her pregnancy when she wants to. Perhaps this can best be dealt with by stating the questions which I am most frequently asked as a gynaecologist and then trying to answer them as clearly as possible.

What can I do to ensure that I never lose my ability to have children?

Of course the short answer to this is 'not much'. On the face of it fertility is something over which we have no control. It is an intrinsic function of the female from puberty to the meno-pause and that function either works or it does not. But that is too facile a statement and there are quite a number of steps that a woman can take to preserve, if you like, her reproductive system in good working order.

From the last chapter we have seen that not only ovulation is required for conception, but one of the other main prerequisites is healthy open tubes. Let us take a look at these two requirements from the point of view of keeping them functioning smoothly.

OVULATION

Frequently the contraceptive used by women before they start their childbearing will be the pill. This acts by preventing the production of ova. There is no evidence that prolonged use of the pill will prevent ovulation resuming once the pill has been discontinued, provided that regular periods and therefore, presumably, regular ovulation, have been present before starting the pill. It is probably inadvisable for someone who has had infrequent periods or who has not had periods for a long interval of time (known as oligomenorrhoea and amenorrhoea, respectively) to use the pill as a form of contraceptive. Although drugs are available to help, it may be much more difficult to restore regular menstruation in such a person, and, more importantly, ovulation, after discontinuing the pill.

So if you are someone who has always tended to have periods which are few and far between be sure that you discuss your contraception with a family planning expert – do not simply ask for, and get, a prescription for the pill from your doctor.

Another point to be made is that there is no proven merit in taking a break from the pill every now and then. Not infrequently the disaster of an unwanted pregnancy occurs in those few months.

And another important point. There is no necessity for the pill to be stopped for a certain number of months before trying to become pregnant. The only benefit in doing so is that it allows one or two normal periods to occur before conception and the resultant calculation of the duration of pregnancy is made more accurate.

To summarise:

1. Prolonged use of the pill should not lessen fertility.
2. There is no merit in having regular breaks from the pill.
3. There is no need to stop the pill for a set time before attempting to conceive.
4. If you have always tended to have infrequent periods with long gaps between, the pill is not the contraceptive for you. Seek expert advice.

OPEN, HEALTHY TUBES

No eggs, however regularly produced, can proceed to fertilisation and transport to the cavity of the uterus when the tubes are unhealthy, damaged or blocked. Figure 4 is a radiograph showing open, healthy tubes.

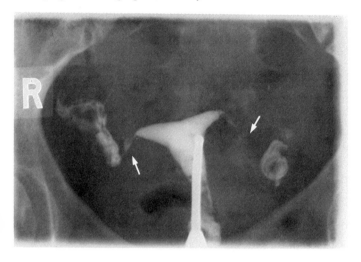

Fig. 4 Radiograph (hysterosalpingogram) showing the open uterine tubes (arrowed)

What causes damage to tubes? If we answer that we can then pick out situations which can be avoided, hopefully conserving the health and well-being of these structures, so vital in the process of conception. Basically, tubes are damaged by infection and that infection may arise in different ways. There are two main situations to be considered.

1. *Infection arising from 'surgical' procedures*: Something like acute appendicitis may lead to secondary infection in the tube and of course no one can be expected to avoid acute appendicitis. But two other situations come to mind. First, the

intra-uterine contraceptive device (IUCD) – loop, or coil. The insertion of one of these into the womb can scarcely be considered as a piece of surgery but for convenience we will consider it under this heading.

There seems to be no doubt that in women who have never been pregnant the use of the IUCD increases the risk of pelvic infection. Not every woman who gets pelvic infection will get blocked tubes but the risk is there and in any case, as we have seen, to function properly the tubes do not just need to be open they need to have undamaged lining cells and unrestricted muscle activity – both of which may be affected by infection.

So it seems clear that apart from some exceptional circumstances the IUCD as a method of contraception is best avoided in the woman who has not yet conceived.

Then the other surgical procedure that carries a risk of pelvic infection, and therefore blockage of the tubes, is termination of pregnancy. An unwanted pregnancy can be a disaster for the woman concerned not only socially but also psychologically. And medically too, it carries its potentially serious implications. Termination of pregnancy is *not* an 'easy little operation', quickly carried out and quickly forgotten. It undoubtedly carries a small but definite risk of pelvic infection. So the message is clear: avoid an unwanted pregnancy, and the necessity for seeking an abortion with its attendant risks, by getting the best contraceptive advice you can and following it faithfully.

2. *Infection arising without preceding surgery*: 'Pelvic inflammatory disease' (PID). Probably the most likely background to PID in the woman who has never had a pregnancy or any intra-abdominal surgery is one of sexual activity from an early age and with multiple partners. It has been estimated that multiple sexual partners may increase the risk of infection more than four times. Obviously a partner

with a sexually transmittable disease is a real risk. Now we cannot really turn back the clock of social and sexual customs, and arguably this is rightly so. But the message is clear: do not enter into sexual relationships lightly or freely. The delight of a moment could have more prolonged, less delightful consequences.

So we have looked at two main prerequisites for a successful pregnancy – production of eggs and open tubes – and considered some of the events that may affect them adversely. There are some other aspects of many people's lives which also need to be considered in relation to future pregnancy. Two things have received quite a bit of publicity in recent years: smoking and alcohol. Let us examine these a little more closely:

SMOKING

Everyone accepts that smoking is a health hazard, but human nature is such that this risk is often ignored. But when it comes to planning a pregnancy most thinking women will want to know more about the dangers of smoking because most will also be aware that there is a risk involved.

Here are some of the facts:

- There is an increased risk of abortion in smoking mothers.
- The babies of women who smoke are smaller than those of non-smokers. And, quite simply, these small-for-dates babies do not thrive so well.
- Prematurity is linked with smoking.
- Studies of stillbirths and newborn baby death rates have shown a rise of significant proportions among the infants of smoking mothers.
- There is some evidence to show that the children of mothers who smoke are shorter in stature and are more retarded intellectually than the children of non-smokers.

And these sobering facts refer not just to heavy smokers – the figures begin to decline after a consumption rate of only five cigarettes per day.

Again the conclusions are inescapable. Smoking is harmful in pregnancy and at all phases of pregnancy. Surely the plan for smoking mothers-to-be should be to give up well in advance of a planned pregnancy, not just to hope that will-power to cut down will be found as pregnancy advances. The harm may already have been done.

As part of a general fitness plan for the older woman contemplating her first pregnancy, to stop smoking is a must.

ALCOHOL

Again there has been a considerable amount of recent publicity on alcohol and its effects on pregnancy and the fetus. In preparation for pregnancy many women will want to know what they should do about their drinking habits. What are the problems involved and should alcohol be totally excluded or simply cut down and, if the latter, to what level?

There is no doubt whatsoever that excessive drinking in pregnancy–what would be recognised by doctors as alcoholism–is associated with severe effects on the fetus. There is a higher death rate among the newborn, and the stillbirth rate is increased. Then in the child who survives there is recognised what is called the fetal alcohol syndrome–and the risk of this may be as high as 30 per cent. What is this 'fetal alcohol syndrome'? First the baby may be born small and indeed may remain stunted. Then other specific features are described: the face may look odd with drooping eyelids, a short up-turned nose, low-set ears and so on; worst of all the brain may not develop normally and mental defect may be present.

This full-blown picture is said to occur in 10–30 per cent of alcoholic mothers. It is estimated as occurring in 1 in 1000 births in northern France, and 1 in 750 births in Seattle,

USA. As yet no similar figures are available for this country but the occurrence of the fetal alcohol syndrome appears to be much less here. But then we reach a difficulty. Most women reading this book are unlikely to be alcoholic by anyone's standards. But most are likely to enjoy social drinking. So what is known about this lesser degree of drinking?

A study in California has suggested that miscarriages in mid-pregnancy occur more often in women taking one or two drinks daily. In New York another investigation suggested that the miscarriage rate was 25 per cent among women drinking only twice weekly. These studies, however, are thought to be inconclusive. Again, other studies have shown an apparent relationship between 'moderate' drinking (e.g. one to two drinks per day equal to, for instance, a pint of beer, two measures of spirits or two glasses of wine) and small underweight babies, with or without some minor physical abnormalities and possibly behavioural problems.

In a recent communication from the Royal College of Obstetricians and Gynaecologists, due acknowledgement is made of the fact that as yet the evidence that moderate or social drinking is harmful to the developing fetus is inconclusive and that many more studies are needed. However, excessive drinking is undoubtedly related to problems of fetal growth and development and it is not yet known at what level drinking can be said to be safe.

Once more the inescapable conclusion must surely be that until more facts are known, alcohol in all but minimum quantity must be regarded as suspect in pregnancy. What better time, therefore, to start cutting down than in the year or two before a pregnancy is planned?

Having dealt at some length with perhaps the most frequently asked question of how a woman can maintain her fertility let us examine some other common queries.

Do my husband's age and health influence our ability to conceive?

The short answer to this one is, up to a point, yes. Here are some of the facts.

A healthy man retains his potency – and possibly his fertility – to a much older age than a woman. But this does not mean that he will necessarily be absolutely fertile. For this his sperm count must remain good. There are many things which affect a man's sperm count and for the purposes of the present discussion it is true to say that to preserve his fertility it is important to retain a healthy lifestyle. Regular exercise, a good diet with avoidance of overweight, minimal or, preferably, no smoking, no excess of alcohol, good genital hygiene and keeping scrotal temperature down by wearing loose underpants instead of tight clothing. Most of this is obvious but it is interesting to know that there is quite good scientific evidence for it.

What about a husband's age itself? It is now thought that the risk of conceiving a baby with a congenital abnormality such as mongolism increases not only with maternal age but also, although to a lesser extent, with the father's age. Some clinics now offer the special test of amniocentesis to check for such abnormalities to women whose husbands are over 55. But it must be stressed that the risk is quite low.

If I am on the pill, how soon should I come off it before starting my pregnancy?

The main consideration here is that if conception occurs soon after stopping the pill and before regular and natural menstruation is re-established it may prove difficult to calculate when the baby is due. With the greater availability of ultrascan – a method whereby the earliest of pregnancies can be shown up on a television screen and measured – this problem is of less importance.

Preparation for pregnancy

It was at one time thought that it was important to allow three clear periods following stopping the pill because it was felt that there might be a relationship between the pill, its effect on vitamin levels in the body and an increased occurrence of neural tube defects (e.g. spina bifida) in the newborn. But the evidence for a link-up is inconclusive and certainly if a pregnancy occurs soon after stopping the pill there is no need to worry. But if you have read about these problems and are at all anxious why not use a simple barrier method of contraception such as a sheath or the cap until two or three natural periods have passed?

Should I have an examination before starting a pregnancy?

I see no real purpose in this. Presumably if you have been under the care of your doctor or a family planning clinic while using contraception of one sort or another, you will have had regular 'check-ups', including smears. If you have previously been healthy then there is no reason to suspect anything that would either hinder you from becoming pregnant or be a major problem in pregnancy.

If, however, being older, you are concerned about a pregnancy, then it is helpful and reassuring to talk to your doctor or to a gynaecologist and ask them all the questions which worry you. Many hospitals indeed are now conducting pre-pregnancy counselling clinics so aware are they of the doubts and anxieties which often affect women approaching their first pregnancy.

As for testing to make sure that you are fertile and able to conceive, this is really an unnecessary and unwarranted investigation. To do it properly would require checking that the tubes are open and this has to be done either by quite a complicated radiographic (*x*-ray) examination or by means of a long narrow telescope, called a laparoscope, which has to be inserted into the abdomen under a general anaesthetic. This is

PROBABLE EGG RELEASE

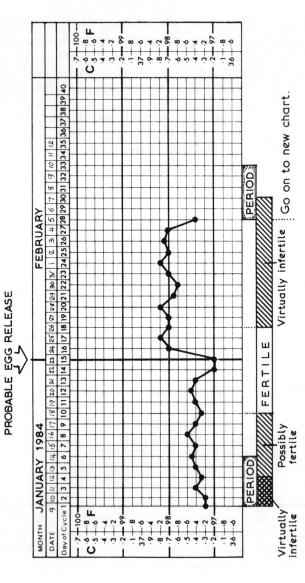

Fig. 5 A basal body temperature chart

scarcely justifiable where no attempt to conceive has yet been made.

Checking whether ovulation is occurring is a much easier thing to do, and if the individual is anxious to know about that fundamental prerequisite of conception there are two simple tests which she can carry out herself without recourse even to medical advice.

THE BASAL BODY TEMPERATURE CHART (Fig. 5)

In the normal cycle where ovulation is occurring mid-cycle, the body temperature is what we call biphasic. This means that at a point about midway through a 28-day cycle for instance the temperature shifts from a lower to a higher level over a space of about 48 hours and the temperature remains at this higher level for the rest of the cycle. Ovulation occurs just before, or during, the temperature change.

The temperature is recorded on an ordinary clinical thermometer (or a special one can be obtained for the purpose) each morning before getting out of bed or drinking tea or similar. The reading is taken after 4–5 minutes and recorded on a special chart, or a piece of graph paper.

To make records like this for three to four cycles will, first, give you an indication of whether ovulation is taking place and, second, when. But let me emphasise that, in my opinion, for a healthy woman who is menstruating regularly to go to even this length in pre-conception preparation is unnecesary and only leads to anxiety.

CERVICAL MUCUS

Another way of checking ovulation and one which is gaining in popularity is self-checking of the mucus of the cervix (neck of the womb). At the time of ovulation the consistency of the mucus changes from being scanty and rather thick to becoming profuse, clear and watery (see Fig. 2, p. 20) and able to be pulled out into a thread. This mucus can be detected by passing a finger right up to the top of the vagina or on to the cervix itself, which feels wet and slippery.

But here again, this is not a test that needs to be carried out obsessively by someone who has not yet given themselves a chance to prove their fertility.

How can I become pregnant most quickly when I want to?

The first thing to be said here – and perhaps the most difficult advice to follow – is not to worry about it. Having stopped contraception then lead life normally, spontaneously and happily, relaxed in the belief that a pregnancy will almost certainly occur sooner or later. The power of the mind on the working of women's physiology is considerable and the achievement of a pregnancy is no exception. Every gynaecologist has the experience of interviewing couples who have been trying unsuccessfuly to begin a pregnancy and arranging investigations for them. But before these investigations can be begun the first period is missed and success has been achieved. Now it is not possible to prove that it was the mental relaxation of knowing that something was going to be done to help which did the trick, but it is tempting to believe so.

So relax, do not get obsessional or neurotic about charts or mucus or anything else.

However, having said that – and admitting that it is more easily said than done – there are a few simple things that can be done to speed up the process. And they all follow from what has been said before. First keep a temperature chart for, say, two cycles only and check when your ovulation occurs. Then you will have an idea for the coming months. Self-examination of the mucus, as described, will back up your interpretation of the chart. Having detected when ovulation is taking place remember that the likeliest time to conceive is on the two or three days around that time. So that is the best time of the month to have intercourse and indeed it is sometimes suggested that intercourse should only take place at that time, on the assumption that the semen will be at its most concentrated and 'potent'. Again this leads to a somewhat artificial aproach to things, losing valuable spontaneity, but if you are getting worried about delay in conception it is, perhaps, worth a try.

If your temperature chart does not give you a clear picture of ovulation, or your periods are irregular, then of course there is a real possibility that you are not producing eggs regularly and it would be sensible to seek help either from your doctor or local family planning clinic or gynaecologist (if you attend one regularly anyway). A simple blood test to measure the hormone progesterone can be done on day 19 of your cycle to check whether ovulation is occurring and if it is not, a useful drug called clomiphene can be given to induce ovulation. This is a drug which is highly successful, easy to take, and very rarely has any undesirable side-effects.

So these are some measures which can be taken if conception does not happen quickly. But above all, let me emphasise again, remain as relaxed as possible about the whole process. Given that your equipment – and your partner's – is in good working order this is probably the single most important piece of advice you can be given.

If I do not fall pregnant quickly how soon should I get medical advice?

I have already indicated that if your periods are very irregular or if, having kept a temperature chart for two or three months, you can see no sign of ovulation then you may want to seek advice. This is perfectly appropriate. However, if you menstruate regularly and if your temperature chart demonstrates a mid-cycle rise you must be a little more patient. The following facts are encouraging:

60 per cent of women become pregnant in the first six ·
months

80 per cent within the first year

90 per cent within eighteen months

These figures refer to women of all ages and it is reasonable to
suppose, therefore, that older women are going to take a little
longer to conceive. In general, investigations for failure to fall
pregnant are begun after a year but many gynaecologists
would be prepared to start investigating the older woman a bit
earlier, although in many ways it would be more rational to
leave it longer!

If I fail to become pregnant what tests will my husband and I have to go through?

First and foremost both partners should be investigated
together, and indeed when seeking advice on delay in
conceiving it is very helpful to the doctor if both are
interviewed together. You will be asked about past illnesses
such as, for the female, pelvic infections, previous abdominal
surgery, acute appendicitis and so on. For the male, mumps
and its genital complications is of chief importance. Then
there are questions about your present state of health, your
mode of life, smoking, alcohol intake and so on. Obviously
there will be questions about your sex life; frequency of
intercourse, difficulties on either side, pain on deep penetra-
tion.

The menstrual history is important and your doctor will
want to know about the regularity or otherwise of your
periods. He will also want to know about which form of
contraception you have used previously. All this provides the
'history' or background of the problem and not infrequently
gives a clue to what the problem is. For example, an acute
appendicitis with peritonitis some time in the past may have
involved the tubes with resultant blockage; or very irregular

periods may suggest lack of ovulation; mumps which had the complication of inflammation of the testicles (orchitis) may diminish fertility in the male (but contrary to common belief this is not a frequent cause of absolute infertility), and so on.

Now to mention the investigations which will be carried out. In the male a simple sperm test will be done. He will be asked to collect a sample of semen, produced by masturbation, into a plastic or glass container which will be provided and this should be done after at least two days of abstinence from intercourse. Some authorities ask that the sample should reach the laboratory within two hours of its production, others would accept longer, e.g. overnight.

What is measured in the semen sample? The total volume, the sperm concentration, the percentage of sperms showing good motility, the normal appearance or otherwise of the sperms; these are the most important features. Many laboratories would ask for a second specimen and certainly if the first shows any abnormalities it is sensible to repeat the test. Some men find it difficult or impossible to produce a specimen under these artificial conditions and in this situation the post-coital test is arranged. Again following a few days of abstinence, the couple have intercourse and next morning, without bathing, the woman attends her clinic and a specimen of the fluid lying in the upper vagina and around the cervix is examined under the microscope. The number and activity of the sperms are looked at and indeed very often the woman is invited to look down the microscope too. It can be a very encouraging experience!

Thinking back over what a woman needs in order to conceive – apart from a fertile male – we can then see what investigations will be offered to her.

First she must produce eggs. We have seen how keeping a temperature chart will be of some help in checking whether ovulation is occurring but it is not as accurate as is required. A simple blood test taken on the 19th day or so of the cycle will be taken and the hormone progesterone will be measured. This is probably the most reliable test for ovulation.

Then the tubes must be open to transport the fertilised egg back into the uterus. (You will remember that the egg is fertilised in the tube (see Fig. 3, p. 24).) There are two main tests used to check whether the tubes are open. A radiographic examination (*x*-ray) called a hysterosalpingogram may be arranged and this can be done either with, or without, an anaesthetic – your gynaecologist will decide. In this test a liquid which shows up on the *x*-ray screen is put into the uterus through the cervix, and if the tubes are open it can be seen on the screen passing into them and spilling out at their ends (see Fig. 4, p. 29). A more recent, and on the whole more favoured, test is to carry out a laparoscopy. This, which we have mentioned before, is a procedure, performed under a short general anaesthetic, in which a narrow telescope (laparoscope) is passed into the abdominal cavity through a tiny (1cm) incision under the navel. A coloured dye is injected into the uterus from below, and through the telescope one can see whether the dye flows through and out of the tubes. A good general view of the uterus, tubes and ovaries – and surrounding structure – can be obtained at the same time. An overnight stay in hospital will usually be advised for this procedure.

These then are the tests – all quite simple – which will be recommended in the investigation of infertility. Depending on their results, treatment will be arranged. It would take too long to discuss the details of treatment for the various problems but very briefly here is an outline of what may be suggested.

1. If the male partner is found to be sub-fertile either surgery to correct an abnormality may be suggested or hormonal treatment by injections or tablets. Simple measures may be advised, such as abstinence from intercourse for a few

days before the fertile period (identified by the temperature chart for instance) so that the semen will be at its most potent at the correct time.

2.   If the ovaries are not functioning then two types of drugs can be used to stimulate them. The simplest is a drug called clomiphene citrate (Clomid), and is taken in tablet form for five days, usually starting on the third day of menstruation. The dosage is regulated by observing the temperature chart for an ovulation response or by checking the level of progesterone in the blood on or about day 19. More sophisticated fertility hormone drugs are given by injection, under close hospital scrutiny with regular hormone measurement. This is something that can only be done in a specialised centre although most larger hospitals with adequate laboratory facilities will undertake it.

3.   If the tubes are blocked then surgery may be offered. Obviously it depends where they are blocked and how badly, and a good gynaecologist will always lay the pros and cons of such surgery before the patient. With the advent of tubal surgery carried out under microscopy the success rate is improved but overall remains much less than one would like.

These then are the facts and it should be clear that a great deal can be done nowadays both to investigate and to treat the couple who fail to conceive within a year of marriage.

It must again be stressed, however, that most older women who are reading this book because they are vaguely worried about deferring their first pregnancy until over 30 years of age, will have no trouble whatsoever in conceiving, usually within a year.

4

Genetic considerations

Every woman, be she younger or older, has a fear of producing an abnormal baby. Much publicity has been given to the subject in recent years so in a book such as this it must receive careful thought. First, some definitions. The word 'genetic' means relating to the origin of an organism and, in the medical context, to the inherited characteristics of a human being.

Now the word 'chromosome'. In the centre of every cell in the body is the nucleus and within the nucleus are twisted strands of material – called chromosomes; and the chromosome plays a fundamental part in the transmission of hereditary characteristics.

Genes can be thought of as like beads on a string distributed along the length of a chromosome and consisting of a substance called deoxyribonucleic acid (DNA) and they are responsible for 'handing on' the properties of the parent cell (Fig. 6).

Every cell in the human body, apart from the egg cells in the female and the spermatozoa in the male, contains 46 chromosomes: 44 are concerned with physical characteristics and are called autosomes; the other two determine the sex of the person. Microphotography can show these chromosomes and the two sex chromosomes have a distinct shape. The smaller of the two looks like a Y and indeed is called the Y chromosome; the other is like an X and is called the X chromosome. In a female, a cell is composed of 44 autosomes and two X chromosomes. In a male, a cell consists of 44 autosomes, one X and one Y chromosome.

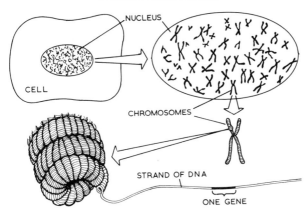

Fig. 6 Cell make-up

Now in the egg cells or oocytes of the female there is a division into two cells, one large, one small. Each contains only 22 autosomes and one X chromosome.

Spermatozoa (or sperm) undergo several changes also and during these changes the number of chromosomes is halved so that a fully mature sperm contains only 23 chromosomes – 22 autosomes and either an X or a Y chromosome. So when a sperm fuses with the large cell of the ovum (the smaller one has no function) it can be seen that the total of chromosomes will be the required 46 – 44 autosomes and two sex chromosomes, either two XX (a female) or an X and a Y (a male) (Fig. 7).

This is how the sex of a baby is determined. Other features are also inherited through the chromosomes – for instance, blood groups.

Now let us come to the problem which worries all mothers, that of congenital abnormalities in their developing baby. We should remind ourselves first that no human being is perfect – everyone, if you look closely enough, has some inherited imperfection, even if it is only big ears or an over-large nose. Having accepted that idea we can think of inherited abnormalities as either minimal, or moderate, or severe.

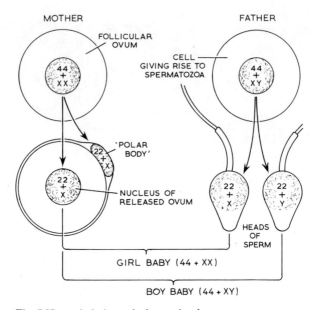

MOTHER

FATHER

FOLLICULAR
OVUM

CELL
GIVING RISE TO
SPERMATOZOA

44
+
XX

44
+
XY

'POLAR
BODY'

22
+
X

22
+
X

NUCLEUS OF
RELEASED OVUM

22
+
X

22
+
Y

HEADS
OF
SPERM

GIRL BABY (44 + XX)

BOY BABY (44 + XY)

Fig. 7 How a baby's sex is determined

MINIMAL ABNORMALITIES

These would include such minor defects as an extra finger, or toe; a small birthmark, and so on. Often these require no treatment although some are dealt with by very simple surgery, often when the baby is a little older. About 1 in every 100 newborn babies are affected.

MODERATELY SEVERE ABNORMALITIES

In this group we, as doctors, would include cleft palate, club foot, congenital dislocation of the hip, abnormalities of the heart. Nowadays these can be corrected surgically allowing a normal existence as the child grows up. Again it has been estimated that 1 in 100 newborn babies show this degree of abnormality.

Genetic considerations

Here we are dealing with a situation which is incorrectable and very often the cause of early death of the baby. Indeed it is important to point out that it has been shown that a number of early miscarriages are of grossly abnormal babies – nature's way of eliminating them. The severe problems which can afflict 1 in 100 newborn babies are conditions such as mongolism, blindness, absent limbs, uncorrectable heart and intestine abnormalities.

What are the causes of these abnormalities? Broadly these are the two groups:

1. What we might call *the intrinsic group*, i.e. within the mother and developing fetus themselves, namely congenital inherited factors. The basic reason for inheriting abnormalities is largely unknown but the study of such problems, known as genetics, has advanced greatly in recent years and if either parent is concerned about the possibility of their offspring inheriting an abnormality, genetic counselling is available, when an expert can discuss and clarify the problem, based on their detailed knowledge of genetics.

The best known example of this group is Down's syndrome (mongolism). Here there are 47 chromosomes instead of 46. Turner's syndrome is the condition in female babies where there is an absent X chromosome. The subject of inherited genetic abnormalities is a complicated one and is beyond the scope of this book. Suffice it to say that if, in planning your pregnancy, you have the slightest concern about a possible inheritable problem then seek the advice of a genetic expert. There are clinics available up and down the country nowadays. The chances are that your worries are groundless.

2. The second group is what we might call *the extrinsic group* – that is abnormalities due to outside factors affecting the baby's development and growth. There is a variety of

factors which can lead to such problems and many of them are very well known nowadays. There is, for instance, rubella (German measles) which can affect the developing baby to varying degrees if the mother is affected during the first three months of her pregnancy.

Then there are x-rays which concern us because although they may not produce abnormalities in the baby they may lead to congenital abnormalities in subsequent generations.

Drugs are a well-advertised cause for concern and gradually a list of drugs to be avoided in early pregnancy, during the crucial formation stages of the fetus, is being built up. Thalidomide is perhaps the best known of all because of the limb abnormalities which it produced. But other more commonly used drugs have been implicated. Some antibiotics are known to cause problems – sulphonamides and tetracycline to name two of the more commonly used.

In general, it is correct to advise that no drug should be taken in quantity or for any length of time in the important early stages of pregnancy. If, of course, a drug has to be taken to maintain normal existence in the mother then this is quite a different matter. Indeed, to stop such a drug would probably cause more harm to the fetus because of the harm it would do to the mother. Taking one or two tablets of, for instance, paracetamol and then finding that you are pregnant is not a cause for concern. It is quantity and duration of treatment that matter – as well as the drug itself. Incidentally, do not forget smoking and alcohol in this context, which we have already discussed.

What then is the risk to the older mother of having an abnormal child? Obviously external factors such as drugs, x-rays or infections affect all age groups alike, although it is possible that the older mother is more likely to be taking medicines. It is the genetic, chromosome-inherited, defects that we are more interested in when thinking about age.

Down's syndrome is well documented as being associated with increasing maternal age. For instance, the risk of such a baby has been calculated according to the age as follows:

> Age 20   1:1923
> 25   1:1205
> 30   1:885
> 35   1:365
> 40   1:109
> and so on until age 45 when it is 1:32.

Other chromosomal disorders increase with age. Between ages 35 and 39 the likelihood that a chromosomal abnormality of any type will occur is approximately 1:70.

Obviously if genetic abnormalities are already known in either the mother's or the father's family the risks are increased.

But the picture is not all one of gloom for a great deal nowadays can be done both to detect abnormalities and to deal with them – not by correcting them but by stopping the pregnancy if this seems the only right and sensible thing to do.

Pre-natal diagnosis of fetal abnormality

As has been mentioned previously many hospitals have pre-pregnancy counselling clinics. Here women and their partners 'at risk' for one reason or another, either because of age or because of having had a previously abnormal child or a close family history of an abnormality, can be interviewed and a reasoned assessment given of their chances of producing an abnormal child. This can be of great benefit to the couple in planning their family.

The methods whereby abnormalities can be predicted are as follows:

AMNIOCENTESIS

Under ultrasound screening (see below) a fine needle is passed through the mother's abdominal wall and into the cavity of the uterus and the water surrounding the baby (the liquor). About 20ml of this liquor is drawn up into a syringe and sent to the laboratory. This test is carried out at about 16 weeks of pregnancy.

What can be learned from investigation of the liquor? A substance called alphafetoprotein may be measured. Many hospitals routinely take blood from mothers at 16 weeks to measure this substance and only if that measurement is raised would the procedure of amniocentesis be offered.

A raised alphafetoprotein suggests the presence of a so-called neural tube defect. This may involve the brain, known as anencephaly, or the spinal cord – spina bifida.

The cells in the liquor may be cultured and the chromosomes looked at. In this way a Down's syndrome baby can be detected. At the same time the sex of the baby can be identified but, incidentally, the parents will not usually be informed of this unless they press for the information. Amniocentesis is not without a small risk of miscarriage – about 1 in 100 – so the procedure is not undertaken lightly or without discussion with the parents.

In general, you would be offered amniocentesis under the following circumstances:

– If you are over 35: or, in some centres, 37 years of age.
– If you have a family history of abnormalities.
– If you have had a previously affected baby.

ULTRASOUND

This technique is widely used in obstetrics nowadays and in skilled hands has proved to be of great value. The basic principle is simply that sound waves are reflected from the interfaces between different tissues, and in the most sophisticated machines now in use the reflected sounds are recorded on a screen as a series of dots of varying whiteness which build up a picture. This picture is so precise on modern machines that shape, size, position and movement can all be assessed.

The uses of ultrasound in pregnancy are many. For instance it can be used to diagnose an early pregnancy and to confirm that it is growing. It is employed in assessing the maturity of a baby, in locating the site of the placenta, in diagnosing twins. And relevant to this chapter, it is of great value in looking for abnormalities of the fetus. In skilled hands, and using the most sophisticated machines the developing baby's brain, spinal column, heart, kidneys and so on can all be examined. It must be emphasised that the procedure carries no risk to the developing baby.

So, linking the last two sections, what usually happens is that in the 'at risk' mother blood is taken at about 16 weeks for estimation of the alphafetoprotein. If this is raised an amniocentesis will be offered and if this again gives a raised alphafetoprotein level a detailed scan can be done to try to locate the site and the extent of the neural tube defect.

FETOSCOPY

This is a newer technique, not available in many centres as yet, whereby a 1.7mm diameter fibre-optic telescope is passed into the pregnancy sac under ultrasound control. Through the telescope the growing fetus can be visualised and pieces of its skin can be taken for laboratory examination; samples of blood from the placenta can also be obtained. Rare disorders of the fetus can be picked up in this way and of course chromosome studies on the fetal blood give a much more certain diagnosis.

The technique of fetoscopy carries its risks to the pregnancy – of abortion or premature delivery. Obviously as it becomes more available a balance will have to be maintained between its benefit in the management of the pregnancy and its risk to the fetus or mother.

TROPHOBLAST BIOPSY

Trophoblast is the name of the cells surrounding the developing embryo and from which the placenta arises (see Fig. 3, p. 24). The inner lining is known as the chorion, and the early embryo, covered by chorion and trophoblast, settles down in, and anchors to, the lining of the uterus by finger-like processes growing out and into the uterine lining (known as decidua). These processes are called villi and a technique has been developed whereby a sample of these trophoblast or chorionic villi can be obtained between eight and 12 weeks of pregnancy, and again the cells can be cultured and chromosome studies carried out.

At the time of writing this technique is only in its comparatively early stages of development but it has obvious advantages in that diagnosis of fetal abnormality can be made earlier than with amniocentesis, ultrasound or fetoscopy.

These then are the methods at present actually available or being developed for the early diagnosis of fetal abnormalities. Along with these methods pre-pregnancy counselling clinics are springing up throughout the United Kingdom and in these the extent to which a couple can be considered to be 'at risk' of having an abnormal baby is estimated and tests arranged after full discussion. No one need accept the tests and everyone should be quite clear as to their value, their validity and their risks.

What if an abnormality is demonstrated? This question will be discussed – or should be – with the couple, *before* investigations, such as amniocentesis, are carried out. If an abnormality is discovered, such as Down's syndrome or spina bifida of severe degree, then the mother will be offered a termination of her pregnancy. This is made clear to the couple beforehand

and they are asked to think about their response. Quite obviously if they will not consider an abortion under any circumstances then there is no purpose in pursuing investigations.

It is, of course, a difficult moral problem. Many people support the philosophy of the 'right to life' and would not condone abortion. Others would emphasise the concept of 'quality of life' and accept the idea of selective abortion for developmental abnormalities.

A couple faced with the decision of what to do about an abnormality will require not only counselling but sympathetic support, and will undoubtedly be influenced by such things as their religion, the severity of the abnormality, previous experience or knowledge of other people with handicapped children.

5

The antenatal period

There are many books available to the pregnant woman, giving her explanations and advice on pregnancy, delivery and the care of her baby (some are suggested on p. 120). No attempt will be made here to repeat these facts, rather we will concentrate on aspects of pregnancy and antenatal care which particularly concern the older mother, and especially the 'first time' older mother. Here it must be emphasised once again that 35 seems to be the age beyond which one is more likely to find problems. It is true to say, however, that in modern obstetrics a woman over 30 will receive extra monitoring in pregnancy, possibly in a special so-called 'high risk' clinic or at the very least her age will be noted by the examining doctor and a careful eye kept on her. 'High risk' clinics have become a common feature of modern antenatal care. What an unfortunate title, however, and it is to be hoped that it is not bandied about in the hearing of those mothers asked to attend them. It is scarcely conducive to the relaxed optimism which should be the aim.

What are some of the commoner antenatal problems found among older pregnant women?

In early pregnancy there is a slightly higher chance of miscarriage and there may be more sickness.

A higher blood pressure is a normal feature of getting older and this may be exaggerated in later pregnancy to give rise to the condition of pre-eclampsia. Under modern conditions this is not dangerous to mother or baby but requires careful management, and admission to hospital for a time will almost certainly be necessary.

Bleeding behind the placenta, pushing it off its attachment to the uterus is commoner in older women. This problem is known as abruptio placentae or accidental haemorrhage and does of course constitute a risk to the baby. This complication occurs more in women over 35 and certainly over 40.

The older woman may have developed certain gynaecological problems which are unlikely in her much younger sisters. The most quoted is fibroids, but here again these benign tumours of the muscle of the womb are found more commonly in the late 30s and early 40s than in the earlier 30s.

Premature onset of labour is commoner in the older ages especially in the primigravida. The risk diminishes with subsequent pregnancies. But let us as always keep things in perspective. Undoubtedly women of 30–35 will, in the vast majority of cases, have a normal pregnancy. Those over 35 will be rather more likely to develop problems of one sort or another and this particularly applies to women over 40. We have mentioned some of the commoner problems but it is worth noting some figures which help to keep things in proportion.

In one reported series of 1500 older primigravidae no problems arose in about 70 per cent, there were higher blood pressure difficulties in about 25 per cent and the remaining 5 per cent had bleeding from the placenta, fibroids or other minor ailments (Fig. 8). But it is the 70 per cent we should concentrate on and it is to be hoped that all older mothers while receiving extra care in pregnancy receive it from doctors and midwives who instil into them justifiable optimistic confidence.

Special features of antenatal care for the older mother

We have already discussed the question of special tests carried out in early pregnancy to exclude abnormalities of development so far as is possible. These will include, if you remember,

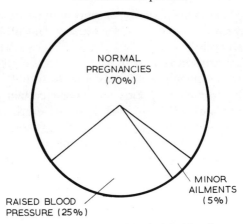

Fig. 8 Diagram showing the relationship of
normal pregnancies in older women to possible
problems

early scanning (often offered to all age groups), the blood
level of alphafetoprotein (again frequently arranged for every
mother), amniocentesis (usually over the age of 37) and
perhaps, in some centres, trophoblast (chorion) biopsy.

These are all special tests. What about routine antenatal
care for the older woman? Very often, because of her age, she
will receive her antenatal care in a 'special' clinic – as we have
mentioned. These are primarily for women with particular
aspects of their present or past health or obstetric history
which warrant special attention in this pregnancy. An older
woman having her first baby would be one such person. One
of the great advantages of such clinics is that generally you will
be seen by the same doctor and very often the most senior
obstetrician of the team looking after you. It would, of course,
be ideal if every pregnant woman could be looked after by the
same doctor throughout her pregnancy, but in the context of
hospital clinics this is simply not possible because of the
numbers involved. A 'team' it has to be, although often that

team will consist of no more than three doctors – the consultant, the registrar and the house officer – so that the individual's chance of getting to know all three is very high.

In a special clinic, women will naturally have more chance of undergoing the various 'monitoring' procedures which are used nowadays to watch closely how the baby is growing and how well its placenta is functioning. So let us look at some of the tests used to monitor baby's growth. The older mother, especially if she is over 35, will very likely have these various tests offered to her.

SERIAL ULTRASCAN

This means that weekly or two-weekly scans are done and measurements of, for instance, the diameter of the baby's head are taken. These can be plotted on a graph which shows the range of normal measurements at the various stages of pregnancy (Fig. 9). Other measurements can be made such as the circumference of the abdomen, the length of the baby's thigh bones and so on.

If a baby does not grow too well for one reason or another this is recognised, and is called either intra-uterine growth retardation or 'small-for-dates'. Several factors are known to be associated with this problem. Cigarette smoking is notorious, and age can also be a factor. Once recognised the situation will be monitored most carefully by scanning and other methods and there may come a time when, contradictory though it may seem, the decision has to be made to deliver the baby early either by caesarean section or by inducing labour. This is quite simply because a stage has been reached when the placenta no longer appears to be able to sustain the pregnancy and the baby is already showing signs of distress, so that it is better and safer for it to be born even if it has to spend its first week or more in a special care baby unit.

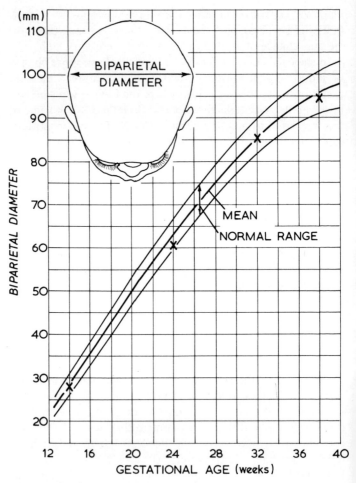

Fig. 9 Ultrascan chart showing measurements of the fetal head

HORMONE ESTIMATIONS

There are certain substances found in the blood or urine of the mother which reflect the function of the placenta, and their levels at various phases of pregnancy have been worked out. To measure these substances, or hormones as they are called, is therefore to measure the function of the placenta and whether it is good and continuing so or not.

Oestriol is the chief one used and may be measured in a 24-hour collection of urine or often (and more conveniently) in a sample of blood. Like serial scan measurements the results can be recorded in graph form and progress followed (Fig. 10).

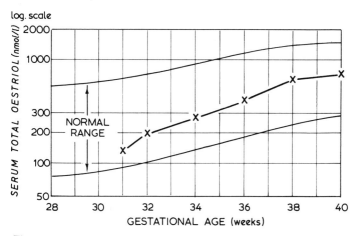

Fig. 10 Graph showing oestriol estimations during pregnancy

Another substance sometimes used as a progress indicator either alone or in conjunction with oestriol is human placental lactogen (HPL).

Neither measurement is worth doing much before 28 to 30 weeks and when they are considered necessary and are started they have to be repeated weekly to make the results meaningful.

FETAL HEART TRACINGS

It is now possible to fix a special microphone to the mother's abdomen and make a tracing of the fetal heart beats. This is often done in the antenatal clinic, fixing the monitor to the mother for a minimum of half an hour. A lot can be interpreted from the tracing – the speed of the baby's heart, the variation between beats (a 'flat' tracing shows a quiet, possibly sluggish and distressed baby) and how the heart rate responds to tightening of the uterus (a 'good' baby will respond by quickening of its heart rate). Figure 11 shows a typical and normal tracing.

These cardiotocograms – so called because they can record both the fetal heart rate and, through another 'microphone', activity of the uterus – are becoming very familiar to mothers in the labour ward but are also quite commonly used in the antenatal clinic.

KICK COUNTS

The mother herself may be asked to count how often she feels her baby kick and to record it on special charts (Fig. 12). Normally with a healthy baby undisturbed by its environment a mother will be able to count up to 10 kicks in an hour.

These are the main methods used in modern obstetrics to monitor special pregnancies where problems may be expected. Never forget though that the basic essential of good antenatal care lies in careful regular examinations, which in turn implies that the mother herself must be willing to attend for examination regularly.

At each examination the mother is weighed, her blood pressure checked and her urine tested. She is then interviewed and examined by the doctor who feels the baby, assesses the

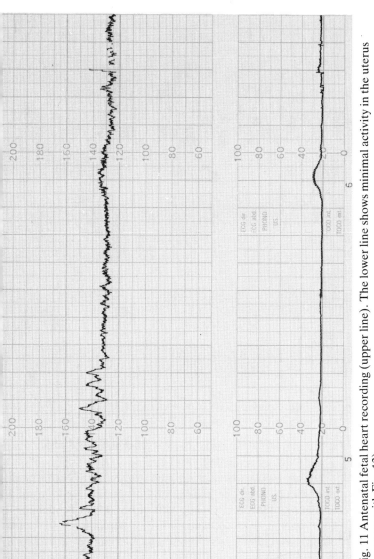

Fig. 11 Antenatal fetal heart recording (upper line). The lower line shows minimal activity in the uterus (compare with Fig. 13)

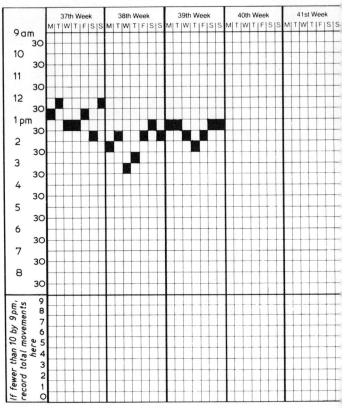

Fig. 12 Fetal kick count chart

way it is lying, whether its head is presenting at the pelvis and so on. All this is routine antenatal care.

In most clinics women are asked to attend every month until they are 28 weeks pregnant, then every two weeks until 36 weeks and then every week until term (which is 40 weeks). The older mother attending a special clinic may be asked to come more frequently than this depending on how the pregnancy is progressing.

Blood tests are carried out at intervals – usually at booking, 28–32 weeks and 36 weeks – or more often if needed, and it has already been mentioned that hormone estimations may be done to check the baby's progress.

These simple aspects of good antenatal care are of fundamental importance and provide the foundation on which electronic or laboratory testings rest. With good care early signs of problems can be detected, the appropriate action taken and complications avoided.

In summary then, remember that the majority of older mothers will have no problems at all in their antenatal period. However, special antenatal care will almost certainly be offered to them in the sense that – depending on age – early chromosome testing by amniocentesis, early scanning for abnormalities may be carried out and later in pregnancy more frequent attendance at the antenatal clinic arranged. Tests to monitor the baby's growth and the functioning of its placenta may be carried out and naturally, if problems arise, admission to hospital will be arranged where even closer monitoring of the baby's well-being can be done. Modern obstetric care is highly technological but the old art of caring has not been lost and sympathy, understanding, discussion and explanation should all be available to the older mother.

6

Labour and delivery

Descriptions of labour and the delivery of a baby are readily available – in books, in films and in antenatal preparation classes. These last, incidentally, provide particular help to the older pregnant mother, which she should certainly make use of. They are available in most centres and allow opportunities not only to hear about pregnancy, labour and delivery but also to ask questions until all doubts and anxieties have at least been thoroughly aired. They are a most useful addition to the services provided for a pregnant mother.

Nevertheless perhaps it would be easier in this chapter simply to go over the main features of labour and delivery, pointing out where events may – or, more importantly, perhaps, may not – be different for the older mother.

There are three stages in labour. The first stage lasts on an average about 12 hours in women having their first babies and about seven in those who have had babies previously. The latent, or relatively quiet, phase of the first stage may last up to eight hours and is not particularly distressing to the mother, but the more active last part of the first stage, lasting three to four hours, is more painful because the contractions are then not only stronger but much more frequent.

First stage of labour

The first stage of labour for the older mother may, on average, take longer. At least this is what is normally quoted in textbooks but in a sizeable number of older primigravidae which I myself studied some years ago there was no significant increase in the number of these mothers who had prolonged labour.

Induction of labour is something which happens more often to the older mother, especially when she is having her first baby. The reason for this is that she is much more likely to have a rise in her blood pressure towards the end of her pregnancy and this is a situation where it is often necessary to start off labour and get the baby delivered. There is no greater reason for the older mother to go beyond her dates compared with younger women but many obstetricians take the view that induction of labour should be carried out rather sooner after term in the older mother than in the younger.

And there are other reasons for the more frequent induction in this group. But again let us keep things in perspective. The older women requiring induction more frequently will almost certainly be over 35 and possibly over 40. The younger of the 'older' group, i.e. 30–35 can expect to behave entirely normally.

INDUCTION OF LABOUR

It may be appropriate at this point to describe the procedure of induction more fully since if it is more likely to happen to you then you will want to know something about it. The word 'induction' literally means to lead into, with the implication of gentleness and lack of force. Many a mother must wonder whether obstetricians have ever considered the derivation of the word induction and as a result a lot of exaggerated stories about the procedure have been spread, among apprehensive primigravidae in particular. Here are a number of straight-forward definite facts about it which may help to paint a clearer and less disturbing picture.

1.   Nowadays no one carries out induction of labour without there being a good reason for it. And modern doctors are well aware of the need to communicate with their patients,

so the reasons for induction should be clearly explained and understood. If not, ask.

2.   In most hospitals now the regime employed is to insert into the vagina a pessary of a substance known as prostaglandin. This has the effect of softening and 'ripening' the neck of the womb (the cervix) and indeed in some cases will actually lead to the onset of contractions and the start of labour. This is often carried out either on the night before induction of labour or in the early hours of the morning.

3.   'Breaking the waters', which is the next step, is really a very simple procedure and if it is done after an epidural anaesthetic has been put in there will be no discomfort whatsoever. If, however, it is done before any such anaesthetic then the discomfort experienced is very little more than with a vaginal examination. The actual breaking of the bag of waters is painless.

4.   Then there is the 'drip' – the intravenous infusion containing the substance oxytocin (Syntocinon). Many women dread this, but there is no need to. With modern equipment the amount of and speed with which the drug is given are regulated to give controlled contractions. If an epidural anaesthetic is being used then an intravenous infusion will always be set up in any case, so that the addition of some oxytocin is a very simple matter.

If, of course prostaglandin pessaries have triggered off labour and it is progressing nicely then there may be no need to use oxytocin at all.

MONITORING IN LABOUR

Monitoring in labour is something which is offered to all labouring mothers nowadays. Very few hospitals are without the necessary equipment but if their facilities are limited then certainly the older mother having her first baby would be an obvious preferential candidate for this valuable technique. In monitoring the baby during labour the mother is strapped to

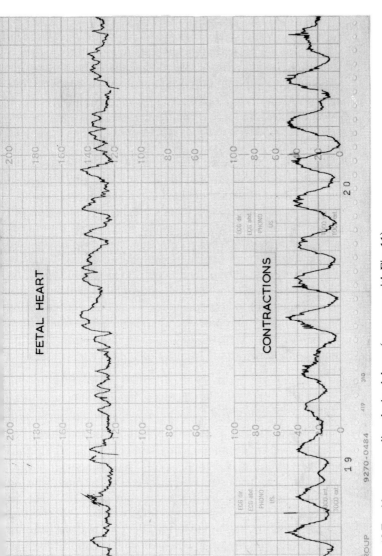

Fig. 13 Fetal heart recording during labour (compare with Fig. 11)

two microphones placed on her abdomen and linked to a recording machine which will produce two tracings (Fig. 13). The top tracing, as we have previously seen, is the beat to beat recording of the baby's heart and the bottom line the frequency and strength of the contractions of the uterus. We can then see how the baby's heart responds to each contraction. Does it get faster? In this case it is described as a good reactive response. Does it get slower? Depending on the timing of the slowing in relation to the contraction this may indicate that the baby is getting truly distressed by labour and that intervention is required to deliver it quickly.

At the time of writing there is some feeling of antagonism against monitoring during labour among a certain group of women who feel that labour should be a natural experience with as little interference on the part of midwives and doctors as possible. One respects their view and of course it is every woman's right to decline fetal monitoring if she so wishes. As an obstetrician I always find it rather strange that women should not want to 'keep in touch' with their babies during labour – after all, this amazing experience of labour and birth is one surely to be shared between mother and baby, not to mention father, who can become quite expert in interpreting fetal heart tracings!

Second stage of labour

Now we come to the second stage of labour, which is the stage when the cervix has completely disappeared, the baby's head descends on to the floor of the pelvis and the mother usually feels the urge to push – *usually*, that is, because with an epidural anaesthetic for instance, that urge may not be present. In that case the second stage will be recognised on examination by the midwife or doctor and the mother encouraged to bear down with each contraction. This is the stage of delivery of the baby and lasts, on an average, one hour in a primigravida and 30 minutes in a multigravida (someone who has had one or more babies previously).

The contractions in the second stage are expulsive and the baby's head is driven downward through the pelvis until it reaches the perineum and then gradually, with each contraction, climbs up the perineum and is delivered. The rest of the baby is born with the help of the midwife or doctor as a result of the following contractions.

In the older mother it is true to say that intervention to deliver the baby is more often required than with younger women. Why is this so and what do we mean by intervention? Certainly in women over 35 it seems that the womb very often does not seem to function quite so well and the contractions during labour are not so effective. There is, as a result, a delay in the opening up of the neck of the womb and in the progress downwards of the baby. The exact reason for this is not clear.

Because of these facts, the second stage of labour is prolonged with sometimes distress in the baby developing and not unexpectedly exhaustion in the mother. Provided the cervix is completely dilated and the baby's head quite well down in the pelvis, intervention takes place in the form of a forceps delivery.

FORCEPS DELIVERY

Many women fear forceps delivery – usually because they have the wrong idea of what is involved. Here is an outline description which tries to tell you truthfully what happens without exaggeration but also without 'covering up' the facts. If the baby gets distressed or the second stage has progressed for some time (e.g. pushing for an hour) without progress then preparations will be made for the forceps delivery. What happens is this – and incidentally, the doctor should explain what is going on: if he does not, ask. Your legs will be put up in stirrups so that there is easier access to the vagina; if you have an epidural no further anaesthetic will be required; if not, an injection of local anaesthetic will be made on either side of the vagina so as to produce numbness of the perineum and lower vagina. Numbness does not remove the feeling of touch so you will be aware of the doctor slipping the two blades of the forceps over the baby's head – one at a time on each side of the baby's head. Then with each contraction while you continue to push you will feel the doctor exerting quite a strong pull. This may feel alarmingly uncomfortable although with the anaesthetic there will be no actual pain, but there is no reason to be alarmed since the forceps act as a rigid cage to protect the baby's head and the doctor's skill will be such that neither you nor your baby will be harmed.

You will have been trained to stop pushing and 'pant' while the baby's head is 'crowned' and passes over the perineum to be born. During a forceps delivery the same is true and the doctor will ask you to stop pushing while he lifts the baby's head out over the perineum. The forceps are removed from the baby's head at that point and the baby's limbs and trunk are delivered normally.

An episiotomy will invariably be required at the time of a forceps delivery, so it would seem appropriate to discuss the question of episiotomy at this point.

EPISIOTOMY

An episiotomy is a deliberate incision into the perineum, made by the midwife or doctor to facilitate the delivery of the baby. Many women think that episiotomies are made without real necessity and the more vociferous pressure groups who are interesting themselves in the conduct of childbirth would claim that they are carried out far too frequently, often in a brutal manner and that they give rise to a lot of long-term discomfort. Let me try to reassure you by giving you the facts:

1. Episiotomies are almost certainly not carried out 'far too often' although the numbers done vary according to the midwives and doctors concerned.

2.   It is quite possible that a long delay before delivery with the baby's head held up on the perineum may give rise to laxity and actual prolapse in later life. So the feeling is that an episiotomy done to expedite delivery *may* avoid this. Notice that I use the word 'may' – this is a problem which has not yet been proved one way or another.

3.   A clean cut surgical incision is more easily repaired, and will heal better than a large irregular tear which is so often the alternative. If a tear seems certain – and some would say it is inevitable in a primigravid mother – then an episiotomy is preferable.

4.   A local anaesthetic is always used nowadays. Either the mother will have an epidural in place anyway or the site of the episiotomy will be infiltrated first with local anaesthetic.

5.   The episiotomy is stitched up after the placenta has been delivered by the doctor or by a midwife trained in the procedure. Naturally there will be some discomfort afterwards. How could an incision in such an awkward part of one's anatomy not be uncomfortable? But this discomfort passes, and long-term problems are very much the exception, not the rule.

CAESAREAN SECTION

Since we have talked about forceps delivery it is appropriate to mention caesarean section next as the older primigravida has indeed got a slightly increased chance of being delivered by this method. Women in their 40s and even later 30s may well plan to make this their only pregnancy and the obstetrician may decide to deliver by caesarean section in the presence of doubt about the capacity of the pelvis and so on.

Other reasons for caesarean section, in all age groups, are breech presentation where the baby comes bottom first (not all breeches will be delivered by caesarean section although the chances of it are much higher in the older woman); where a baby is showing signs of distress before labour, the so-called 'light for dates' baby; medical conditions in the mother such as diabetes or even a tendency to diabetes, which can develop in some mothers during pregnancy; a low-lying placenta; a pregnancy which goes beyond term and where induction of labour fails or is thought inadvisable. And there are many other reasons for the operation.

What happens with a caesarean section? In summary an incision is made into the mother's abdominal wall (usually a so-called bikini incision, which explains itself) and down through the various layers to display the uterus. The uterus is then opened through a transverse incision in its lower part, or 'segment' as it is called and the baby, followed by its placenta, is lifted out of the uterus. The uterus and abdominal wall are then repaired in layers.

Caesarean section is a surgical procedure, and one must expect the discomfort of an abdominal wound afterwards. But there are several ways of minimising this by pain-relieving drugs or continuing the epidural for 24 hours after delivery and the mother is often surprised at how quickly she can move about quite early afterwards. The operation may be done under a general anaesthetic or, frequently nowadays, if both mother and father request it, an epidural may be used so that the mother is awake at the delivery and her husband can sit with her. Naturally, precautions are taken so that neither husband nor wife need witness the actual surgical procedure!

EPIDURAL ANAESTHESIA

We have mentioned epidural anaesthesia several times and although descriptions of this procedure will be found in books describing pregnancy and labour perhaps it will be useful to mention it briefly here. There is no doubt that in most maternity units the older primigravida will be encouraged to accept the idea of an epidural. Very often, indeed, there will be a medical reason for advising it and hypertension (high blood pressure) is the condition which comes to mind in the case of the older woman. An epidural anaesthetic is very effective in keeping the blood pressure down during labour.

In brief, an epidural anaesthetic consists of an injection in the back under local anaesthetic and a fine polythene catheter passed into the so-called extra-dural or epidural space in the lumbar region of the backbone. A local anaesthetic is injected through the catheter so that the sensory (pain) fibres of the spinal nerves supplying the uterus, vagina and vulva are temporarily numbed. The motor (movement) fibres of the spinal nerves will be affected too but to a lesser extent so that as well as losing the sensation of pain the mother may well feel her legs to be very heavy and be unable to move them. Mothers may find this a bit disturbing but remember that the effect is only temporary and permanent paralysis does not occur.

The insertion of an epidural is not painful although some uncomfortable sensations may be experienced. Its advantages are many. It allows greater relaxation of the mother during contractions and because fear and the inevitable 'tightening up' reaction to pain inhibit the progress of labour, labour can progress more quickly and smoothly which is obviously much better for the baby (and its mother and father!).

One worry which mothers have is that with an epidural anaesthetic in place they will have no urge to push in the second stage and therefore there will be a greater need for forceps delivery. This is to some extent true but in recent times there has been a move towards not encouraging the mother with an epidural in place to push whenever the second stage is reached but to allow the natural forces of the uterus to push the baby downwards provided that its condition remains entirely satisfactory. When the epidural lightens and the mother gets the sensation of wanting to push she is then encouraged to do so.

PAIN RELIEF IN LABOUR

Having discussed epidural anaesthesia in some detail we must not forget the more traditional methods of pain relief in labour. These are still in use and the commonest is the drug pethidine given as an intramuscular injection. This is useful in relieving moderate pain and particularly for women who have prepared themselves to cope with pain through breathing exercises practised in their antenatal preparation classes. As an adjunct to this, pethidine in small but repeated doses can be invaluable.

Then there are the inhalational methods, chiefly the use of the Entonox machine which delivers a mixture of 50% oxygen and 50% nitrous oxide. The mother will be taught how to use the machine and, therefore, to administer the mixture herself; its greatest use is towards the end of the first stage and during the second stage. It, too, may be a useful addition to the effect of pethidine.

Third stage of labour

Now we come to the third stage of labour. This is the phase between the birth of the baby and the completed delivery of the placenta and membranes. The delivery of the placenta is usually helped by the attendant midwife or doctor and lasts from 5 to 15 minutes, and is completely painless. This part of labour should occur perfectly normally in the older mother. It is theoretically possible that if her first stage has been prolonged by a rather 'inert' uterus – and perhaps this has been followed by a forceps delivery – the uterus will not clamp down quickly after delivery and extra blood loss will result. But in fact a drug, ergotamine maleate (Syntometrine), is almost always given by intramuscular injection at the time of the delivery of the baby's shoulders and this encourages firm contraction of the uterus afterwards thereby minimising bleeding.

And if the first stage has been slow an intravenous infusion with Syntocinon will almost certainly be in place and this can simply be speeded up to help firm up the uterus.

So in this chapter we have briefly considered the three stages of labour and pointed out aspects which may be different for the older mother. Once more it hardly needs to be stressed that the majority of older mothers will start labour spontaneously, will go through labour without incident and deliver their babies with perhaps only the help of an episiotomy. Modern management of labour is efficient and skilful. The preparation of the mother for labour remains, however, of prime importance and every mother – especially the older – should take the opportunity of reading, of listening to authoritative teaching, and above all of asking questions.

7

After delivery

The period of time, usually taken as four weeks, which follows the delivery of the baby is called the puerperium. During this time the changes which have taken place not only in the uterus but also in other parts of the body – the vagina, the breasts, the blood flow and so on – gradually return to normal. As one would expect, there have also been considerable emotional changes during pregnancy and in many ways these are enhanced in the few days immediately following the birth of the baby. The feelings of happiness, awe, excitement and perhaps a tinge of nervousness that flow over the mother when she first sees her baby cannot really be described in any book. They are individual and personal to each mother. It is not surprising therefore that mothers often become a bit 'blue' about the fifth day following delivery. This is especially true of the older mother. The pent-up excitement and apprehension of pregnancy are abruptly over, the delivery may have had something of an anti-climax about it (especially if a caesarean section has had to be performed) and now the business of getting to know this new being as her own is suddenly here. Joy and fulfilment are the main emotions but, after a few days, worry about feeding, about handling the baby, about ability to cope, may flood in to supersede the other feelings and a kind of depression may occur. This may be made worse if breast feeding is proving difficult, if sleeping at night is poor, and if relatives and visitors overexcite and overtire the new mother.

But remember that this 'depression' is a completely normal occurrence, much less obvious than the picture I have painted, and may be very transient indeed. Every midwife and doctor knows that it can occur and is ready to support and understand. So if it happens, do not worry or feel guilty if a feeling of disinterest towards the baby is part of the picture – it is all quite normal and it will pass, to be replaced once more by the initial feeling of happiness. These are times when an understanding, supportive partner can be of such help and, especially in the case of the older mother, to read books about pregnancy together, to attend preparation classes which have a session or two for fathers also and to talk through fears and phobias with one's partner are all of the greatest help.

It has already been mentioned that the perineum will inevitably be quite uncomfortable and this may last for several days. But there are applications which can be used for relief of such discomfort, and certain simple pain-killing (analgesic) tablets will help while not upsetting the baby if you are breast feeding.

The main aspect of the puerperium which may affect the older woman, pregnant for the first time, is breast feeding and its successful establishment. Antenatal preparation classes and books will have taught a lot about it but it is often more difficult to put these things into practice. Unfortunately it is true that successful breast feeding is more difficult to establish successfully in the older woman. But again let us keep things in perspective. I am referring to women in their later 30s, even early 40s and of all women who are just over 30 the majority who wish to, will breast feed successfully.

Every encouragement will be given to the mother, for all midwives and most doctors are dedicated to breast feeding. But remember, if breast feeding cannot be satisfactorily established then bottle feed without guilt or qualms, for in the all important business of the baby bonding with its mother, contentment and a relaxed happy atmosphere are the key notes – not exactly induced by a hungry frustrated baby struggling at the breast of a tearful, tense and miserable mother.

You will learn about breast feeding during your antenatal period but some points to help, bear repeating.

1.   Remember that the milk does not fully 'come in' until the third or fourth day. The baby will be put to the breast meanwhile as his suckling helps to stimulate the process of milk production but do not worry if he gets very little.

2.   See that the baby gets on to the breast properly – and the nurse will help you here – so that he does not 'chew' on the nipple and make it sore. Cracking of the nipple is both painful and risky, in that it allows an entry point for infection. So it should be avoided if at all possible.

3.   Cleansing of the nipple area both before and after feeding is important.

4.   It is easy to say, but be as relaxed as possible before feeding and sit comfortably, holding the baby securely and in a comfortable way.

5.   Drink plenty of fluids and above all do not worry.

Bonding of mother and baby is discussed a lot nowadays, particularly by paediatricians who recognise how important it is in the future development of the baby. Now the mother who has a normal delivery, who holds her baby immediately after delivery and maybe even puts him to the breast right away starts the bonding process at once. It is, of course, a mutual process – baby to mother, mother to baby (and don't forget father to both mother and baby if he is, hopefully, present at the delivery) – and develops fully with the establishment of breast feeding. We have seen previously how more frequently the older mother may have to be delivered by forceps or even by caesarean section and also we have to remember that problems such as 'small for dates' babies may occur more commonly in the older mother. All these mean that not infrequently the baby has to be under special care from the moment of delivery, possibly even in an intensive care baby unit. This separation of mother and baby is unfortunate but will only happen where it is really necessary. Often a photograph of the baby is given to the mother very quickly so that she has it by the bedside – no real compensation, admittedly, but better than nothing. And as soon as the mother is able she will be taken to the nursery to see her baby, to handle him if that is possible and begin to help to nurse and care for him. She will be encouraged to express her milk and then helped to feed the baby with it as soon as possible. Bonding in this situation is not so direct or immediate but it takes place and indeed the bond between such a mother and baby when he finally emerges from the nursery, now strong and healthy, is often all the stronger.

These then are some of the aspects of the puerperium which may particularly affect the older woman. One thing is clear to me as an obstetrician. All women, but especially the older first mother, need plenty of rest and a good deal of what we in the medical profession call 'TLC' – tender loving care. Rest is difficult in a busy maternity ward but is not impossible and certainly visiting times should be adhered to with a limited number of visitors for the first few days being encouraged, and, incidentally, to stay a limited length of time! TLC will be given by the staff within the limits of their time and duties but can be given in large measure by, first, the husband or partner whose prime task this must surely be, and secondly by the new mother's own mother or a close female relative. Supportive partners and a relative or two go a long way to smoothing out the puerperal path.

And finally, do accept the idea of staying in hospital for a week or 10 days if this is your first baby. You will be surprised how strange and nervous you feel when you first go home so take advantage of the opportunity of rest, meals prepared for you, regular hours and supportive staff around you which the maternity unit provides.

When you do go home your own doctor will be informed and a health visitor will visit shortly after your return from hospital. She will help with any problems and may particularly be of value with the continuing feeding regime of the baby.

The postnatal examination

This subject is also fully discussed in books about pregnancy (see p. 120) but perhaps it is reasonable to add a comment or two here in so far as it relates to the older woman. Most older women having been anxious about achieving a pregnancy, about passing through pregnancy safely and emerging with a healthy normal baby are on the whole more anxious about whether they have returned to normal afterwards than are younger women, who have regarded the entire process much more as a matter of course. Many hospitals no longer provide postnatal clinics as such, simply because so few women attend – which adds validity to my last comment. General practitioners, however, will carry out postnatal examinations and, of course, if you have attended an obstetrician privately an examination six weeks after the birth will be arranged. If you feel strongly that you would like your hospital doctor to see you postnatally then make this request while you are in hospital and most doctors would arrange an appointment, understanding your anxieties. Certainly if your delivery has been a complicated one, ending, for instance, with a caesarean section or if you had some problem such as hypertension during your pregnancy a postnatal examination will be arranged for you.

What happens at a postnatal examination? Apart from asking how you are and how the baby is thriving the doctor will want to examine you. First, the breasts, to make sure that they are healthy. Then he will feel the abdomen and finally carry out a pelvic examination to ensure that the uterus has returned to normal.

Some clinics carry out cervical cancer smear tests at the postnatal examination – others will do them at the booking clinic.

Finally, and most importantly perhaps, you will be given advice on the future based on an explanation of what took place in this pregnancy, the delivery and so on. You will get an opportunity to ask questions and it is often advisable to have these written out so that you won't forget to ask certain things. Thus, for instance, 'Why did my blood pressure go up during pregnancy?' 'Is it normal now?' 'Will it go up in another pregnancy?' Or 'Why exactly did I have to have a caesarean section?' 'Will I have to be delivered by caesarean section next time?'

The thoughtful obstetrician will usually have answered most of your questions during or after his examination but he may not always think of every point which you would like clarified. So ask. Finally contraception, the aspect of a postnatal examination which many would say is the most important of all. Not only advice may be given but prescriptions for pills or fitting of intra-uterine devices or measurements for caps can all be organised at the same session. The question of contraception will be discussed in Chapter 9.

8

Sundry questions

In this chapter I will try to pick the questions which, in my experience, are asked most frequently by the woman who is having her first baby at a rather older age. I am tempted to leave several pages blank at the end of the chapter for the many other questions which I will undoubtedly miss and for which you will be seeking an answer from your own doctor! (Such blank pages will be found following the index.)

The present pregancy

DELIVERY AT HOME

A lot of women feel, quite understandably, that they would like to have their babies in their own home. After all, what better environment for a baby to enter – quiet, no fuss, husband there, familiar surroundings and so on?

But there are potential risks, of that there is no doubt. There is no need to list them but in general let me point out that a first pregnancy and labour are truly untried events – there is no previous experience to base them on. It seems to me only common sense, therefore, to have your baby safely, in surroundings where help is immediately at hand, where the baby can be monitored continuously and all the back-up facilities of specialist support for both you and your baby are available. If something goes wrong at home you then have to face transfer in labour to hospital or even a 'flying squad' emergency call to your home – sure a most alarming experience.

Sundry questions

Nowadays, in spite of pressure on the part of some women who would disagree with what has just been said, there are very few doctors who would willingly agree to a first baby being born at home, far less the first baby of an older woman.

CAN MY OWN DOCTOR LOOK AFTER ME?

The answer is, yes. But the sensible thing is for your own doctor to share responsibility for your care with the hospital specialist. This is, in fact, known as 'shared-care' and what happens is that you visit your own doctor at regular intervals, carrying with you a card into which are written the findings at each examination, and then at salient points in the pregnancy you attend the hospital clinic. These times are usually at the beginning of pregnancy (after it has been confirmed by your doctor) for 'booking' when a full examination is made, your social and medical details recorded, and the preliminary blood test taken. Thereafter the hospital usually likes to see you at between 28 and 32 weeks, at 36 weeks and then each week until term. I say 'the hospital' advisedly because you will usually not see the same doctor on each occasion although your records will always be in front of the examining doctor, which does provide some continuity of care. This variation in attendant doctors is a source of great consumer criticism and indeed obstetricians are aware of its drawbacks. But in the context of a maternity unit delivering for example, 2500–3000 babies each year and therefore running clinics for 50 or more women it is obviously impossible that one doctor should undertake all the antenatal examinations. Not only is it impossible but I do not actually consider it to be safe.

A 'team' of obstetricians is usually made up of the consultant, the most senior and experienced person; his assistant, a registrar or senior registrar; and his senior house officer, who is the most junior member of the team and very much in training. When the house officer is considered able to he sees his own patients. It seems sensible surely, that the women seen and examined by him, should be given the opportunity on other visits to the clinic to be seen by either of the more senior members of the team. In this way every woman has the chance of meeting, being examined by and discussing her progress with, the more experienced obstetrician. In the event most women get to know the members of the team well and the idea that you will see a different doctor each time is an exaggeration.

In many present-day maternity units, as has already been mentioned, the older woman in her first pregnancy will be looked after in 'high priority' clinics and there she will almost always be seen by the same doctor, namely the consultant, often in the company of his senior assistant, the registrar.

WOULD I BE BETTER TO ARRANGE PRIVATE CARE?

The advantages of private care are that you are indeed looked after by one person – and that person is of your choosing (helped usually by your doctor). You get a greater feel of individual attention and when you have your baby your private obstetrician attends the birth personally. Under the health service the midwife is your attendant and will deliver baby if everything proceeds normally. (The trained midwife is particularly expert at delivering babies but if anything goes wrong she will immediately send for medical aid.)

Then after your baby is born you will, naturally, be provided with much more privacy (a single room) and luxury – most modern private maternity units are beautifully and comfortably furnished. This is something which a general National Health hospital cannot possibly provide.

Are there any disadvantages of having a baby privately? The first and obvious one is the expense. This varies according to the hospital and indeed, the consultant. (There are no 'fixed' fees in private medical practice.) If you are considering having your baby privately then you would be well advised to find out about fees first. Under certain special circumstances your medical insurance company (if you have a medical insurance) may be prepared to assist, but again you would be well advised to find out where you stand in this respect before embarking on what can be a very expensive exercise. No one wants a crippling series of hospital and medical fees to cloud what should be one of the happiest events of her life.

Modern private maternity units are well equipped in respect of baby monitoring, laboratory facilities, operating theatres and special after-care of both mother and baby. It was not always like this and this is where private obstetrics came in for a lot of criticism. It is still sensible for you or for your own family practitioner to check your local private facilities.

National Health care in this country may be basic in terms of individual attention, of comfort, of privacy but it has all the facilities of modern obstetrics aimed to deliver to you a healthy normal baby and it provides a team of experts to look after both of you. And it is free. This is something which can be matched by very few other countries in the world.

WHAT HAPPENS AFTER I GO HOME WITH MY BABY?

There is quite a vogue at present for mothers to go home after delivery, if not after a few hours then after 48 hours. Arrangements are then made for the domiciliary midwife to visit her at home and keep an eye on both mother and baby. But in my opinion a woman who has just had her first baby, especially if she is older and even more especially if she has been trying for a long time to have that baby, should remain in hospital for a minimum of seven days. It takes all of that time to feel strong again, to feel comfortable so far as the perineum and stitches are concerned, and most important of all to get to know her baby, to feel at ease handling it and bathing it and so on and, of course, to establish feeding, be it breast or bottle. When you return home you will notice at once how strange and insecure the outside world seems after the care and security of hospital. This is quite natural as is the feeling of uncertainty about coping with your new baby.

It is often a good idea to have your mother or mother-in-law (if liked, as the recipes say) or some female relative, preferably with experience of babies of their own, to stay with you and help for a time. If this is not possible then certainly your partner should take time off work for at least a week and preferably two, to be at home to help and support you when you return from hospital.

Your own family doctor will be informed by the hospital when you are discharged. So your doctor may visit you soon after you get home and certainly the health visitor will call, as we have seen.

All your questions about exercises, the care of your stitches, how much activity and domestic work you should undertake and so on should have been answered in the hospital by the midwife or by the obstetrician. There are many excellent books about pregnancy and after available to mothers now, and most of your questions will be answered there. All of these apply to the older as well as to the younger mother. Because of the natural extra anxiety of the older mother it is important that she should read about it all.

The matter of an actual postnatal clinic has already been raised. The older mother probably needs to be reassured more than the younger woman that everything is back to normal. Your own doctor may well carry out postnatal examinations, which are very simple, as we have seen, or if not, then request that you should be seen in the hospital clinic. You are unlikely to be refused when you explain your anxiety.

Incidentally, all these comments apply equally to the mother who has been delivered by caesarean section. In her case she may well be in hospital for 10 days at least. Otherwise progress is similar and her activities on return home will be very little more restricted.

IF I WANT TO RETURN TO WORK HOW SOON SHOULD I DO SO?

This depends on the nature of the work. It is certainly inadvisable to return to work under six weeks following confinement. Paid maternity leave, when it is granted, includes 11 weeks after the birth which is some guideline. It is better to seek advice from your midwife, doctor or obstetrician on this point because of individual variation. Again in the case of the woman in her late 30s it is sensible in general to take a little longer before returning to work, giving plenty of time for restoration and getting to know and care for your baby. But there is enormous individual variation not only in response to childbirth but in the wish to return to work quickly afterwards.

And there must be many more questions which the older woman wishes to ask. Often they will be asked by all ages of women, and so this book should be read in conjunction with books dealing in general with pregnancy and the puerperium. Any other questions – and their answers, of course – could be jotted down at the end of this book (after the index).

Perhaps the most important question of all is to be answered in the next chapter – contraception.

9

Contraception for the older woman

Most modern women, younger or older, are interested in contraception – family planning, in other words. Every thoughtful couple wants to space their children not just for financial reasons but for emotional and other personal reasons. So the need for good but safe methods of contraception is obvious.

This is another subject which is well covered in books and in pamphlets and most women reading this sort of book will almost certainly have been under the care of a family planning clinic, their family doctor or a gynaecologist for this very reason. After her first baby the older mother may well wish to review her previous method of contraception, so it is perhaps useful to look at the different methods available and make particular comment on each in relation to age.

Lactation and contraception

Since we have left the question of contraception to the end of this book, following the delivery of the baby, it seems logical to think about the lactating, breast-feeding mother, whether she requires contraception and if so, what can she safely use.

Breast feeding has been claimed to be the best method of contraception available. This is not entirely true and indeed in Western countries it must never be relied upon on its own as a method of birth control. Suckling stimulates the production of a hormone called prolactin and this hormone prevents ovulation. But the production of prolactin depends on frequency of suckling and it has been shown that breast feeding as a method of contraception is much more successful in societies where breast feeding is frequent and prolonged – not well spaced out as in Western societies.

So whereas the lactating woman is relatively infertile she must never be encouraged to consider herself absolutely so. This particularly applies to the older woman who may not lactate so successfully or for so long. A method of contraception suitable for use in conjunction with breast feeding must be considered.

As we consider other contraceptive measures, mention will be made as to whether they can be used while breast feeding is continuing.

Hormonal contraception – the pill

This remains the most successful method of contraception available. When we speak about 'the pill' we refer to the combination of the two hormones, oestrogen and a progestogen (that is a progesterone-like compound). In the new mother who is breast feeding the 'combined' pill is not a suitable method of contraception because the production of milk may be inhibited. In this situation the so-called 'mini'-pill, which contains only a progestogen is ideal. One of the problems – if not the only one – of the mini-pill is irregular bleeding and the lactating mother is unlikely to experience this. Together with the relative protection of breast feeding, the mini-pill is a good method of contraception, at this time.

Most authorities still feel that when women are over the age of 35 it is better to stop the use of the combined pill. But this attitude is changing, and the feeling is more and more that if a woman is not obese, if she does not smoke and if she has a normal blood pressure she may remain on the newer low-dose pills over the age of 35. Two important comments must be made here. First, it has been clearly shown that heavy smoking (15 cigarettes or more per day) is as important as, if not more important than, age. For example, a heavy smoker of under 30 is running as big a risk of thrombosis and related problems from the pill as a non-smoker of between 35 and 39. The message is loud and clear. If you want the convenience and security of the pill with minimal risk to health, stop smoking or keep it to an absolute minimum.

The second comment that must be made is appropriate at the time of writing. Whether it remains appropriate at the time of publication remains to be seen.

Two articles have appeared in the medical journal, *The Lancet*, linking certain pills with cancer of the breast and of the cervix. The relationship was broadly with long-term use before the age of 25 of combined pills containing a higher 'potency' of progestogen, which was somewhat arbitrarily assessed. The feeling, however, remains – and has been stated categorically by that watchdog of prescribing, the Committee of Safety of Medicines – that the conclusions of these papers are not as yet acceptable, but that it nevertheless follows that the lowest dose of both oestrogen and progestogen which is effective, should be used. It is unnecessary to add that regular examinations to include breast examination and cervical smears, must be carried out on all women using the pill.

The progestogen-only pill (mini-pill) is suitable for older woman and overall has a much lower incidence of side-effects of all kinds with one exception. This is not a health hazard but carries a high inconvenience rating–irregular bleeding. Periods may be so erratic on the mini-pill that it becomes unacceptable. If there are no such problems, however, the progestogen-only pill can be continued right up to the menopause.

The intra-uterine contraceptive device (IUCD)

This can be a very useful method of birth control for the older woman. She (and her medical attendant) may remain unhappy about the pill in spite of apparently logical and convincing arguments and statistics. If the device causes no problems it can be forgotten (apart from regular checks), and is effective. Troubles in the form of unacceptably heavy periods, infection and so on mean that it may have to be removed but it is certainly worth trying as the next step, when for one reason or another the pill is discontinued.

Its insertion in the nursing mother is easy and is usually done at the six-week postnatal examination. If you have been delivered by caesarean section you may find that your doctor prefers to wait for eight or even 12 weeks after delivery before inserting the device.

There are several different types of IUCD now available but the most used (and most effective) contain copper, which seems to add to their efficiency.

The barrier methods

These basically consist of either the cap (or diaphragm) used by the woman, or the sheath (or condom) used by the male. They act, as their name suggests, by creating a barrier between the sperm and the female reproductive tract. Used carefully on every occasion they are reasonably successful and have had a resurgence of popularity. They are particularly useful for married couples who have evolved a more 'regulated' life – less so for young, uninhibited 'spontaneous' couples.

Their chief advantage lies in the fact that they are what is called 'non-invasive'. In other words, no chemical is being added to the bloodstream and no 'foreign body' is being left for any length of time inside the body. This is a considerable attraction to many women.

After childbirth the cap is not very convenient until after the six-week postnatal period when healing, and therefore comfort, of the perineum has taken place. The sheath, however, may be useful during this time, certainly to improve the contraceptive effect of lactation.

With the barrier methods the use of spermicidal creams is advised. Using creams or foams alone is not really effective.

Newer forms of vaginal caps and barriers are becoming available. The cervical cap has been available for some time and proves very successful for some women – more acceptable than the bigger vaginal cap. Sponges of polyurethane impregnated with spermicidal cream are now being introduced. These have the additional advantage of being able to be left in place for several days.

For the older woman, worried perhaps by the continuing adverse publicity of the pill or perhaps with health reasons for not using it, and unattracted by the IUCD or with a history of infection which would contra-indicate it, turning to the barrier methods, particularly the diaphragm, and learning their use carefully has a lot to commend it.

The safe period

This method relies on recognising when ovulation occurs. This is unreliable to say the least, although many women committed to this method of birth control become adept at identifying ovulation. It can be shown by maintaining a temperature chart for a few months and seeing when the significant temperature change tends to occur (see Fig. 5, p. 36). Changes in cervical mucus may be detectable by some women – scanty and 'dry' immediately after menstruation, profuse at the time of ovulation and thick and sticky before menstruation (see Fig. 2, p. 20).

The method requires a lot of thought, and study of the individual cycle. It also requires a lot of self-control. For couples who are older, who have had just one baby and who do not mind how quickly another pregnancy occurs it may have its uses. It is the method officially approved by the Roman Catholic Church.

Sterilisation

This book has been written for the older woman embarking on her first pregnancy. A lot of what has been said also applies to the mother who may have had one or more pregnancies under 30 and then after a gap becomes pregnant again when she is in her late 30s or even into her 40s. The question of sterilisation as a method of contraception particularly applies to her.

Either the woman or the man can be sterilised. It is an unfortunate word, with its implication of something totally bereft of vitality and attractiveness and it is a pity that doctors both continue to use it and make no real attempt to replace it with an equally precise but less chilling word.

In the male, it is a vasectomy, which means division of the small duct (the vas) which runs from the testicle to the prostate gland and thence to the penis – the canal for the passage of the sperms in other words. It is usually an outpatient procedure carried out under local anaesthetic and complications are very few.

For women, the operation of sterilisation involves blocking the Fallopian tubes by one method or another. It may be done by an 'open' operation – that is, a small incision is made into the lower abdomen under a general anaesthetic and the tubes are either tied or removed altogether. Perhaps the commoner method nowadays is by using an instrument called a laparoscope, which is a very thin long telescope. This is inserted through a tiny incision at the lower border of the umbilicus and through it the uterus and the tubes can be identified. Another instrument – a long, even thinner, forceps – is passed into the lower abdomen through a 'nick' in the skin and, visualised through the telescope, it is used to grasp each tube in turn and to place either a tiny clamp or silastic ring over a segment of it. This is a very simple operation in the hands of an expert and usually only necessitates 24 hours or less in hospital.

Two things must be said about sterilisation. The operation must be regarded as final. There are procedures to reverse the operation but they are not very successful and not widely available. So if a couple are contemplating sterilisation they must be quite sure that they want to take this final step. Then at the opposite end of the scale there is a failure rate to the operation – perhaps 1 in 1000 for female sterilisation, less for the male procedure. For some reason re-canalisation of the tubes occurs and a pregnancy may result.

One other important point to remember about female sterilisation. It does *not* alter the woman in any way – she goes on menstruating, she looks the same, she does not reach the menopause sooner, her libido remains as before. In fact, if a 'final' method of contraception is really wanted and the relatively inconvenient alternatives discarded, sex life can become much more relaxed and enjoyable.

Now how does sterilisation fit into the plans of an older woman? If she has just had her first pregnancy it is unlikely that she will want to be sterilised. Some women, however, in their late 30s, married perhaps late to a man who may already have children whom she looks after, do request sterilisation after one baby. This is quite understandable but it is always sensible to wait for at least a year to be sure that the baby is growing and thriving satisfactorily. Older women who already have children and whose most recent baby resulted from an error or failure of contraception are ideal candidates for sterilisation.

These then are the main methods of contraception available. There are others – injectable progestogens, 'morning-after' pills, to mention two. These are not yet satisfactory and will not be considered further here. For the older woman the choice is really as for the younger, especially if she is under 35. And there seems to be no need abruptly to stop the pill if it suits her, the moment she reaches that age.

Abortion

It seems pertinent to discuss this topic briefly in a book such as this. Although the abortion law has been in action since 1967 there are still a lot of wrong ideas in people's minds about the question of abortion. By definition, abortion is the termination of a pregnancy before the end of the 28th week of pregnancy. The law states quite clearly under what categories a pregnancy is allowed to be terminated: 'If

1. the continuance of the pregnancy would involve risk to the life of the pregnant woman greater than if the pregnancy were terminated;
2. the continuance of the pregnancy would involve risk of injury to the physical or mental health of the pregnant woman greater than if the pregnancy were terminated;
3. the continuance of the pregnancy would involve risk of injury to the physical or mental health of the existing child(ren) of the family of the pregnant woman greater than if the pregnancy were terminated;
4. there is substantial risk that if the child were born it would suffer from such physical or mental abnormalities as to be seriously handicapped.'

Abortions not conforming to these categories are still illegal – and this is not always appreciated by the general public. There is not an 'abortion on demand' service in this country. Many women feel that there should be and their arguments may be valid but so far doctors must adhere to the law in reaching their decision about an individual's request to stop their pregnancy.

The operation is most easily carried out under 14 weeks of pregnancy. A general anaesthetic is usually given and the pregnancy removed by suction curettage of the uterus. Later pregnancies can be terminated using a different method – usually by injecting a drug called prostaglandin into the uterus via the abdominal wall or through a catheter passed through the cervix. A miscarriage is thereby induced.

The later pregnancy may also be terminated by a full abdominal operation known as a hysterotomy. This is really a caesarean section in miniature and is not so frequently used nowadays since the advent of prostaglandins.

Perhaps this description of abortion makes it sound easy and trouble free. Regrettably it is not. Problems such as haemorrhage and damage to the uterus can occur at the time of the operation, haemorrhage and infection may occur in the following few weeks and, more worrying, chronic infection, blockage of the tubes and sterility may result in the long term. In the author's opinion it is not an operation to be asked for, or agreed to, lightly.

Where does abortion fit into our discussion about the older woman? It may be that the professional woman of over 30 has decided not to have a family and then through an error or natural failure of contraception, finds herself pregnant. Not infrequently she then seeks abortion, possibly on the grounds of age. From what we have said previously this does not constitute a legal reason for abortion on its own, for with modern obstetric care age is no bar to pregnancy and delivery of a healthy normal baby – as I hope is now obvious.

Or we may find the older woman with an established, perhaps already teenage, family who finds herself unexpectedly pregnant. Very often her immediate thought is to have an abortion. But with help and counselling she may decide to continue with the pregnancy – and almost always this 'Benjamin' brings the greatest happiness to the family. Of course, the family which is already experiencing financial

96

strain would genuinely find it impossible to look after another child and feel that the stress imposed on the existing children would be too great. Such a woman may have real grounds for abortion but in my experience she requires a lot of thought and counselling – not just an 'off-hand' agreement to stop her pregnancy, as she may have considerable regrets afterwards.

A great deal more could be written about this emotive subject over which there is still a lot of controversy. Suffice it to say in relation to this book that age alone is neither a legal nor necessarily a sensible emotional reason for abortion.

10

The partner's role

This chapter is primarily intended for the men. Hopefully, many will have read, or at least glanced through, the preceding sections so that already they will be aware of what concerns and worries their partners. Perhaps they have even talked about these things together and shared their understanding of the answers to their questions. Some of what has been written was directed at the potential father – pre-conception factors, male aspects of inheritance, male infertility and so on. But in this chapter I aim to discuss quite a different aspect of male involvement and although much of what I say may well be quite obvious nevertheless it will do no harm, and possibly some good, to put it down in writing. I want to consider the role of a true partner, a 'significant other person' as one writer has referred to, in the support of a woman both physically and psychologically before, during and after her pregnancy, and, in particular, the older woman embarking on her first pregnancy.

Preparing for pregnancy

It goes without saying that the decison to embark on a pregnancy should ideally be a mutual one. Laying plans together, anticipating the beginning of a true family and planning for the longer term future all bind a couple together even more closely. Individuals' circumstances vary widely and deferment of a pregnancy may be necessary, but where the woman is already in the later 20s, and especially the early 30s, undue deferment is not really sensible. So the career-orientated male, intent on not only establishing that career thoroughly but in having his ideal house, car and, indeed, lifestyle as well, before 'allowing' his partner to contemplate a pregnancy, should think again and try to take stock of medical, physiological and psychological factors. This is especially so if his partner is longing to have her first baby, is anxious about problems if she leaves it too late and increasingly feels unfulfilled.

The other side of the coin is seen quite often too – the woman is deeply involved with her career and has no immediate intention of pausing in her progress to bear children. Her partner may be quite anxious to have a child but she is not – yet. In either situation the decision may become not a pleasurable one to be made together but a source of irritation and mutual resentment.

As a gynaecologist my advice would be to consider each others' feelings in the matter very carefully, discuss it often, lay plans and maintain your sense of mutual anticipation.

When the time comes to start a pregnancy, and, especially if the couple is older, it may be that reassurance will be sought, especially by the woman, not only by reference to books such as this one, but by visiting a general practitioner or specialist gynaecologist. Both partners should try to attend such a consultation together. Not only does a woman in this situation find the presence of her partner reassuring and supportive but also four ears are undoubtedly better than two and what one misses the other will have understood. Afterwards mutual discussion can take place with great benefit.

What a man can do to preserve his own 'fitness for conception' has already been mentioned. His lifestyle, weight, drinking habits, and smoking should all be critically looked at and the loving supportive partner will ensure that his style of living will do nothing to increase anxieties.

The antenatal period

A man's role during his partner's pregnancy is of tremendous importance. Several points come to mind and there are others.

First, it is of the greatest benefit if he learns about and understands the process of pregnancy. He can read books about it – preferably sharing them with his partner – and in many antenatal preparation classes nowadays at least one 'husbands also' session is held and he should certainly attend. He will have the opportunity at that time not only of having his own tutorial but also of meeting other men in the same situation, of sharing experiences and ideas, and above all of asking questions of the experts. I would also recommend that, wherever possible, he should come with his partner to her antenatal clinic visits – to see and hear what is going on and, above all, to share the experience with her.

If it is not really possible for you to give up the time undoubtedly required to become so closely involved then at the very least remain interested in your partner's progress throughout pregnancy. Remember that she may be worried, she is almost certainly a little apprehensive of what is happening and to get her to talk about it, to ask her questions and to share in her feelings goes a long way to give her a feeling of support and reasurance. Above all never forget that as her pregnancy grows many women feel ungainly and unsightly; so reassure her by paying loving attention to her: open admiration when it is called for, will go a long way to increase her self-confidence. Continue your mutual social activities throughout pregnancy and encourage your partner to look, and therefore feel, her best.

Some of my comments at this point must be directed at the woman who, hopefully, will read this chapter even if it is not directed at her primarily. Every pregnant woman should remember that however happily and mutually she and her partner have made the decision to embark on the pregnancy once it is obviously growing she will inevitably become absorbed by it. But this can lead to some exclusion of her partner without her realising it. It behoves her, therefore, to make a conscious effort to remain loving and caring in her attitude to him, to keep her appearance attractive and refreshing to look at and, above all, to involve him in everything that is going on but without becoming a pregnancy bore! Encourage him to join you at antenatal clinics wherever possible and this is, I believe, particularly important in the case of our older mother who, as we have seen, will almost certainly be receiving extra care and monitoring. To understand these things together can be very reassuring. Incidentally one of the most exciting antenatal investigations to share is the ultrasound scan. Actually to see your baby together for the first time even only as a white outline on a television screen is a very emotional moment for most couples and ought to be shared.

Labour

It is in labour that a man can play his greatest and most supportive role. The months of waiting are over; perhaps they have culminated in a few weeks of increased anxiety for the older couple when blood pressure may have risen and even hospitalisation may have been necessary. When labour begins every support and encouragement must be given to the anxious mother and who better to give it than her partner?

Most men nowadays want to be present in the labour room and all modern maternity units actively encourage this. A few men do not want to be there throughout labour and certainly not at the actual delivery. This must be respected and no pressure should be brought to bear on him (by staff or spouse) to change his mind. A queasy, fainting partner is of little help to anyone. But this is where proper mutual antenatal preparation – by books, by classes, by discussion – can be of such help.

During labour take an interest in what is happening – the cardiotocogram machine and its recording is of particular interest to most men – and above all radiate calm and confidence to your partner. If you do not understand what is going on, ask. Above all do not get 'hyped up' and transfer your agitation and anxiety to your labouring partner.

Encouragement, mopping of her brow and so on are of great importance in the second stage when the true meaning of the word labour comes into force. When the baby is born your partner will want to hold it right away. This is a moment for you both to savour and your mutual feelings cannot be described in a matter of fact book like this. It is customary for the baby to be taken away for cleaning and dressing and for the male to be ushered from the labour room while any stitching that is required is carried out. I would like to suggest that you quietly and politely stay where you are – beside your partner – and, indeed, if the baby is still in the labour room this is a good and valuable opportunity for you to hold and cuddle the baby yourself. After all he is yours and bonding between you and him is just as important as between him and his mother. Bonding of all three together is of even greater importance.

The postnatal period

Your own – and your partner's – feelings at the moment of your baby's birth may be quite disturbing – they may be a confused mixture of elation, apprehension and not infrequently a feeling of anti-climax. This is all quite normal. At this moment particularly your partner will welcome your strength and support, your overt affection and your tacit sympathy for what she is undoubtedly feeling. She is obviously tired, elated of course, but this is moderated by all she has just gone through.

A particular word of advice at this point. If on delivery your baby needs resuscitation because he is not immediately breathing too well he will be surrounded by paediatricians and nurses all attending to his needs – and very expertly too, nowadays. As the father, do *not* raise a fuss and ask questions and create confusion however much you would like to. I have seen this happen with very undesirable results. Leave the experts to their job, stay with your partner and give her all the courage, strength and support which she needs. And this same comment is equally valid for events during labour. If problems arise let the obstetrician do his job unhampered; there will come an opportunity soon enough to ask questions, although you will almost always be kept in the picture by the staff in these days of better medical communication.

Then come the days following delivery. Your partner will be tired, she will almost always suffer a 'reaction', and 'fifth-day blues' are a very real entity. It is at this point that she may become unduly fatigued, feel a sense of anti-climax, feel nervous and edgy, sleep badly and become quite irritable if not down right irrational towards her partner and others. However difficult, accept this as normal and remain calm. Do not add to the situation by burdening her with domestic and other problems and above all try to remain patient and never join her in quarrelling and anger. It will pass, often in a day or two. If you are worried seek an opportunity to speak to the ward sister or doctor. Often it is valuable for them to have their attention drawn to a state of affairs which they may not have noticed.

Getting overtired is one of the reasons for this depression episode and so after the birth it is often a good idea for you to become the regulator of visitors. Of course she will want her close relatives – mother and sisters, for instance – to see the baby soon after delivery but tell them not to visit in numbers and certainly not to stay for long with the new mother at first.

When the day arrives to bring the new baby home the father's role becomes even more important. However impatient your partner may have been to leave the hospital she will find life strange and uncertain to begin with after she has left the safe and supportive surroundings of the maternity ward. Try to arrange to have a week or more off work to be with her, and however undomesticated you may have been previously there is no reason why you should not have given yourself a crash course in domesticity while your partner was in hospital and so be ready to take charge at home. On many occasions a female relative or friend may be available to come and help for a week or two. This is of course an ideal arrangement.

Continue to take an interest in the care and management of your baby. Learn how to handle him, bath him, change his nappies and particularly be prepared to share the burden of getting up at night to attend to his needs. In this way you will remain close to your partner, you will relieve her of a lot of fatigue which can be so harmful to mutual pleasure in this novel situation you now find yourselves in and above all you will get to know your baby and he you.

A piece of advice for the women reading this chapter. Almost all men feel a bit threatened by the arrival of their new baby. This is normal. They have not really been able to share the experience of pregnancy however hard they try and certainly not the experience of birth although being present in the labour room from start to finish helps a lot. So justifiably they feel that now they will have to share their partner's love with the baby and assume that they will be the losers. This can have a profound effect on some men. The new mother should be aware of this and by word and action set about reassuring her partner otherwise. It is true to say that when marriages run into later difficulties not infrequently it is because the mother devoted her time, her energies and her interest almost exclusively to her children and her partner was presumably expected to accept this and play his part as best he could. Beware of this, right from the start, from the moment of your baby's birth.

Finally a word about sexual intercourse. During pregnancy this can continue without risk but naturally the man will want to be particularly gentle with his partner. If, however, there is a problem such as a threat to miscarry or late bleeding or a risk of premature labour then intercourse may be inadvisable. You should be told about this under such circumstances but if in doubt, ask.

In the postnatal period there is no hard and fast rule about when intercourse can or cannot be resumed. The perineum will be too painful at first especially when a large episiotomy has had to be made. By the six-week examination this has usually healed comfortably and intercourse can take place thereafter without difficulty. Some couples prefer to wait longer, others make love successfully before this time without any problem.

Remember the need for contraception even in the early weeks of the puerperium and even if breast feeding. This has been discussed elsewhere. It behoves a man to be particularly sensitive to his partner's natural fear of falling pregnant at this time. This applies especially to the older mother who may have had problems in her pregnancy and possibly in the delivery of her child and who should be given plenty of time to enjoy her first child without being plunged into a further pregnancy too quickly.

11

The newborn baby

Any couple with sufficient interest to buy – and read – a book such as this when planning their pregnancy will doubtless add to their library when conception occurs. And at least one of the books on their reading list will be on the care of the newborn baby. A chapter such as this may therefore seem unnecessary but it has been inserted to round our discussion off, as it were. All mothers feel somewhat apprehensive about their new babies and it has been said that the older mother is even more so. I am not sure how true this is but I do believe that having been concerned about the whole question of pregnancy, labour and delivery at a later age the older mother is naturally particularly anxious first to know that her baby is normal and healthy and then to be sure that she keeps it that way!

So in this chapter I propose only to outline the features of a normal newborn baby and to touch on some things which the new mother may find worrying or difficult to cope with. Obviously greater detail must be obtained when the time comes from bigger more comprehensive books and, much more importantly, the advice, reassurance and help of midwife, health visitor, paediatrician and family doctor – all there to help you – sought whenever necessary.

The normal baby at birth

Your baby will be examined at or soon after birth and this detailed examination will usually be carried out by a paediatrician – a doctor specialising in baby and child care. Try to be present when your baby is examined. It is immensely reassuring to see each system being checked in sequence – and found to be perfect.

The head circumference may be measured and the size and tension of the fontanelles assessed. The fontanelles are the spaces between the skull bones, the larger being at the top of the head near the front.

The eyes are not normally open and will certainly not be forced open to be examined.

The mouth will be examined, the doctor putting his little finger in to feel the palate and to make sure that it is completely developed.

The baby's heart and lungs will be listened to with a stethoscope.

His abdomen will be felt gently and the external genitals inspected. In the case of a male baby the testicles will be felt for to see whether they are both down in the scrotum.

At this point the doctor will pick the baby up and turn him over. This is to feel the spine and make sure that it is symmetrical and normally developed.

The opening into the bowel, the anus, will be felt gently to be sure that it is open.

Finally the limbs will be inspected. Fingers and toes will be counted, the feet and their alignment checked and the hip joints tested for any evidence of instability or actual dislocation.

These are the medical steps in examining the newborn baby. The doctor should, and will, if he is asked, explain what he is doing as he is examining the baby.

From the mother's point of view – a lay point of view – there are one or two points to be made about the baby's appearance. The baby's general appearance will be the first thing that strikes you. At birth he tends to be dirty, covered in vernix (the white cheesy coating that babies have on their skin) mixed with blood. When he has been bathed and dressed he looks much better and you will probably – and rightly – assume that he is the loveliest baby you have ever seen. But just occasionally you will not think any such thing and you may be quite disappointed with your baby's looks. This is quite a normal response as some babies do indeed look quite ugly until they are a few weeks old. If you become worried about any feature do not just keep your fears hidden – air them, ask questions, however foolish you may feel, and be sure to get satisfactory answers.

Another aspect of your baby's appearance which may concern you is his skin, especially the skin, and colour, of the fingers and toes. This may be wrinkled and wizened looking and bluey-white in colour. All quite normal and will improve in a matter of days.

The first week

If it is your first baby and particularly if you have had anxieties about having him at all because of your age, you would do well to stay in the maternity ward for at least a week. The attraction of going home early is considerable but you will quickly appreciate the security and expertise which hospital offers you. If you have a problem the midwife is immediately on hand and if she cannot deal with it the doctor is readily available. After all this time of waiting surely one week of assisted 'training' as it were is entirely sensible.

First *feeding*. 'Breast is best' as we all know and establishing breast feeding is something which we have already discussed. But if for one good reason or another it is to be bottle feeding then you will be taught to prepare feeds, how to sterilise the utensils and so on. What about the timing of feeds? It has rightly been said that clocks and scales play a major part in the routine of the new mother in hospital. This is true and of course it can be modified once she returns home – but to begin with some sort of routine is helpful.

For most babies four-hourly feeding will prove satisfactory although smaller babies may need three-hourly feeds. If feeding on demand is preferred it very quickly establishes itself to a three- to four-hourly routine. These timings refer to both breast and bottle feeding. In the case of breast feeding the time given to the baby at each breast is quite short at first but quickly extends – to about 10 minutes each side by about 10 days.

Details of feeding are beyond the scope of this book but they are learnt very quickly by the mother encouraged as she is by the midwife and later by the health visitor.

Then *crying*. To the new mother particularly after she has left hospital, the crying of her baby can be a very real concern. What does it mean – pain, too cold, too hot, colic, attention seeking or what? A mother soon gets to know the reason for her own baby's cries and learns how to deal with it. Many differences of opinion are offered as to how to contend with the crying baby from 'always pick him up' to 'leave him to have a good cry'. As usual the answer lies somewhere between. If he is hungry or thirsty then satisfy his needs, if he is cold then see that he is cuddled and then settled down with warmer coverings; if he is wet or dirty change him; if he is just grumbling before sleeping (everything else seems all right) then leave him for a little and he may well settle. Colic after feeding can be a real source of worry to the mother. Learn to wind your baby properly during and after feeding and particularly at the end of the day. Discuss the problem with your health visitor or family doctor if necessary.

Bowel problems can also worry a new and inexperienced mother. The looseness or firmness of the stool, the colour of the nappies, soreness of the buttocks can all be a source of concern. Again detailed understanding of these points can be obtained from larger books, and by asking, not so much other mothers (although a trusted friend with a young family can be a great source of help) but the health visitor or general practitioner. The occasional loose greenish stool is normal – frequent loose, watery, green stools which are offensive are not and should lead you to seek medical advice. The occasional rather firm crumbly stool may be normal – persistent hard dry stools are not and again advice should be obtained.

Skin rashes in babies are quite common. Scratching of his face should be avoided by keeping nails trimmed and by wearing mitts. Heat rashes are common especially in the armpits and groins. Lighter clothing will help. Nappy rash is one of the commonest problems. It is caused by ammonia which results from substances in the urine. Frequent changing of his nappy is necessary and your doctor will prescribe some simple cream to use after washing the baby. Sore buttocks can be treated quite simply by exposure.

Respiratory tract infections in newborn babies can be a source of great worry to the parents. Colds and snuffles are not uncommon and the usual precautions of keeping him in a warm environment, clearing his nose of excess mucus and giving him extra fluid is usually all that is necessary. If his breathing becomes laboured you may well need to get medical help. As an immediate aid to the baby's breathing boil a kettle in his room so that the air is kept moist.

There are many other problems to be met with in the new baby. But mostly they are entirely minor and of no lasting consequence to the baby. If you are in doubt, however, do seek help.

Tables 3 and 4 list two other aspects of baby care which

seem to concern women a lot. Remember the timetable of baby development (Table 3) is not a railway timetable so your baby may not be exactly 'on time' each step of the way. This is quite normal. The immunisation programme (Table 4) is a sugested one but your own doctor or local clinic will advise you further.

Table 3. Milestones of development in the first six months

Month 1	Automatically grasps with fingers Lying prone – may momentarily lift chin off mattress Seeks out nipple: sucks: swallows: cries Sleeps a lot
Month 2	Lying prone – lifts head up repeatedly Smiles Eyes focusing and follows moving objects
Month 3	Lying prone – holds shoulders and head off mattress Tries to grasp objects
Month 4	Plays with his hands Turns his head towards movement or noise Laughs Plays with rattle
Month 5	Full head control Able to grasp objects
Month 6	Rolls from prone to supine position Grasps his feet Begins to laugh at simple 'play' Begins to show likes and dislikes of foods

Table 4. Programme of immunisation

Age	Vaccine	Interval between injections	Notes
Birth	Tuberculosis (BCG)		Only to babies at high risk
3 months	Diphtheria, pertussis (whooping cough), tetanus (triple antigen) Poliomyelitis (oral vaccine)		Diphtheria and tetanus only if pertussis vaccine contra-indicated
4½–5 months	As above	6–8 weeks after 1st dose	As above
8½–11 months	As above	4–6 months after 2nd dose	As above
12–15 months	As above	At least 3 weeks after 3rd polio dose	
5 years	Diphtheria and tetanus Poliomyelitis	At least 3 years after basic course	
10–13 years (girls)	Rubella (German measles)		
11–13 years	Tuberculosis (BCG)		If tuberculosis test negative
15–19 years	Tetanus poliomyelitis		

Finally I have not commented on what happens if you have twins, if you have a premature baby or if you have an abnormal baby. Twins – or more – are a handful to say the least and learning to look after more than one baby from the start can be a time-consuming task. This is where the help and support of your partner are particularly invaluable – not to mention the help of health visitors, relatives and friends.

A premature baby may well have to remain in hospital for some time. If it is not to be too long you may well want to stay too. If he is in the special care baby unit (SCBU) you will be encouraged to be with him as much as possible and to help nurse him and handle him wherever possible. All this helps bonding which otherwise would be difficult.

To talk about an abnormal baby here is inappropriate simply because, of course, there are too many abnormalities to think about. Hopefully if your baby has a problem it is a simple one which can be dealt with medically or surgically – congenital hip dislocation, cleft palate and so on. The management of this sort of problem – and even more so if the baby does not survive – is primarily, in my opinion, in the hands of the medical and nursing staff who by their skill, honesty and devotion should be able to help the mother and father concerned to understanding, courage, acceptance and hope.

12

Epilogue

The aim of this little book has been to examine the doubts and fears of the older woman facing a pregnancy either for the first time or, unexpectedly, after a lapse of time. It has been directed chiefly at the first of these. It is to be hoped that many of the questions which trouble such a woman have been answered but I am sure that many remain unanswered. Space has been provided at the end of the book into which I suggest you enter other questions which you are still not sure about – and, more importantly, the answers to them. Pregnancy, delivery and, above all, the puerperium when you find yourself alone with your new baby, are times of natural emotion and anxiety – it would be strange if it were not so – and to be able to refer to your notes must go some way to relieving tensions and worries. Seek answers to your questions not only by reading but above all by asking the experts – your midwives, your obstetrician, your family doctor.

In this way you will get maximum enjoyment from the experience of childbirth and that most precious of possessions, your own son or daughter.

Glossary

abruptio placentae (accidental haemorrhage)   Bleeding which follows the premature separation of a normal placenta

alphafetoprotein   A substance measured in either blood or liquor. A high level may be associated with a neural tube defect (see below), e.g. spina bifida

amenorrhoea   Absence of menstruation

amniocentesis   The procedure whereby a fine needle is introduced through the abdominal wall into the amniotic sac surrounding the fetus to obtain a sample of the fluid. It is used in antenatal diagnosis of some congenital defects, e.g. spina bifida

anovular cycle   A menstrual cycle without the release of an ovum

autosomes   The non-sex chromosomes. There are 22 pairs

breech   The word used to describe the situation when the baby's bottom is coming into the pelvis first – rather than the head which is the more common finding

caesarean section   From the Latin *caedare* – to cut. The operation of incision of the abdominal wall and muscle wall of the uterus (womb) to allow the fetus to be delivered

cardiotocogram   A record of the fetal heart beat

cervical smear (Papanicolaou smear)   The scraping taken from the cervix to enable the cells to be examined for early signs of cancer

cervix   The neck of the womb (uterus)

chromosomes   The paired threads of DNA (see below) in a cell nucleus which carry the genetic code. There are 46 chromosomes – 22 paired autosomes (see above) and 2 sex chromosomes – X and Y (see below)

clomiphene   A drug used to stimulate ovulation. The trade name is Clomid

contraception   The prevention of a pregnancy by physical or chemical methods

corpus luteum   The structure which remains after the egg has been shed from its follicle

decidua   The thickened lining (endometrium) of the womb during pregnancy

differentiation   The specialised development of structures from cells enabling the distinctive features to be recognised

DNA   Deoxyribonucleic acid. It is in the form of long strands (a double helix) which contain the essential genetic components. It forms the chromosomes

Down's syndrome   More familiarly known as mongolism

endometrium   The lining of the womb. In pregnancy the fertilised ovum is implanted into it

epidural   A procedure whereby local anaesthetic is injected into the extra-dural space of the spinal column. It produces pain relief in labour

episiotomy   An incision made into the perineum under local anaesthetic so as to enlarge the exit for the baby

fetal alcohol syndrome   A collection of signs in the *baby* which are associated with heavy consumption of alcohol by the mother. Stunted growth and mental retardation are not uncommon

fetoscopy   A recently developed technique whereby the growing fetus can be visualised directly via a fine telescope passed into the pregnancy sac

follicle   The living structure(s) in the ovary which contains the ova (eggs)

FSH   Follicle stimulating hormone. It is produced by the pituitary gland and stimulates the growth of the egg-containing follicle in the ovary

gene(s)   A unit of DNA responsible for a person's inherited characteristics

gland   A structure which produces fluid or chemicals

hormone   A chemical substance produced by a gland. It influences distant structures by being carried to them in the bloodstream

HPL   Human placental lactogen. A substance secreted by the placenta during pregnancy. One of its functions is to prepare the milk-secreting cells of the breasts for the action of prolactin (see below)

hypertension   High blood pressure

Glossary

hypothalamus The part of the brain lying above the pituitary gland. One of its functions is the control of menstruation

hysterosalpingogram A special radiograph (*x*-ray) which shows whether or not the tubes are open

hysterotomy An opening into the uterus to allow the evacuation of a fetus. It may be used in the event of a late abortion

IUCD Intra-uterine contraceptive device. 'Loop' or 'coil' are other names used

laparoscope A slender telescope-like instrument which is inserted through a tiny incision of the abdominal wall to allow the abdominal or pelvic organs to be viewed directly

LH Luteinising hormone. It is produced by the pituitary gland and stimulates the development of the corpus luteum (see above) and hence the production of progesterone (see below)

liquor The fluid filling the pregnancy sac in which the baby floats

menopause The time of the last menstrual period

menstruation The monthly period or flow of blood from the vagina

morula One of the early stages in the development of the fertilised ovum

neural tube defect A defect in the development of the spinal cord leading to congenital abnormalities, e.g. spina bifida. It may be diagnosed antenatally by amniocentesis (see above)

nucleus The central body of the cell containing the chromosomes. It is surrounded by cytoplasm

obstetrics The science and art of caring for, and delivering, pregnant women

oestriol A type of oestrogen (see below). It is the weakest of the three and is really a breakdown product of oestrone

oestrogen The female sex hormone manufactured in the ovary; during pregnancy it is produced in the placenta. There are three types: oestradiol, oestrone, and oestriol

oligomenorrhoea Infrequent menstruation

ovary The female organ which contains eggs and produces the female hormones, oestrogen and progesterone

ovulation The shedding of an unfertilised egg (ovum) from its follicle

ovum (pl. ova) Literally, an egg. It refers to the egg which is released

pelvic inflammatory disease (PID) An inflammatory condition affecting the organs of reproduction. If an acute infection of the tubes is allowed to become chronic there is a likelihood of the tubes becoming non-patent thereby preventing fertilisation of the ovum

pituitary gland A ductless gland situated at the base of the brain, producing hormones which influence menstruation, ovulation and lactation

placenta The organ which develops in pregnancy linking the fetus with the mother allowing absorption of nutrients into the fetal blood and elimination of waste into the maternal blood. The placenta is delivered as the third stage of labour

pre-eclampsia A rise of blood pressure occurring in pregnancy with protein in the urine. Sometimes called pregnancy-induced hypertension

primigravida A woman having her first pregnancy

progesterone The second of the female hormones produced by the ovary. It prepares the womb for pregnancy. Progesterone is also manufactured by the placenta

progestogen A progesterone-like substance

prolactin A hormone from the anterior lobe of the pituitary gland. It stimulates lactation

prostaglandins A group of drugs with an effect on the cervix and uterus, nowadays often used to stimulate the onset of labour

puberty The transition of a child into a young adult

puerperium The period between childbirth and the time when the womb has returned to its normal size, about six to eight weeks

rubella German measles. A mild infectious disease caused by a virus. The virus is capable of crossing the placenta hence the risk of deformity occurring in the fetus

semen The fluid ejaculated by the male at orgasm, containing spermatozoa

smear See cervical smear

sperm Spermatozoa (see below)

spermatozoon (pl. spermatozoa) The male reproductive cell which is produced in vast numbers in the testicle and released by ejaculation

trophoblast The name of the cells surrounding the developing embryo from which the placenta arises

Glossary

'tubes'   Fallopian or uterine tubes. The two hollow tubes which project out from either side of the upper part of the uterus. These tubes end in finger-like processes, the fimbriae, which over-hang the ovaries and pick up the eggs produced on the surface of the ovary

Turner's syndrome   A condition found in female babies where there is an absent X chromosome

ultrasound   A method using sound waves to produce a picture on a screen (for instance, of the uterus or ovaries or fetus)

uterus   The womb. A hollow pear-shaped muscular organ lying within the pelvis. Its cavity is lined by a special tissue, the endometrium. If pregnancy occurs, the fertilised egg becomes implanted into it

vasectomy   Male sterilisation. Part of each vas deferens, the tubes which carry the sperm, is excised

X chromosome   The sex chromosome which is *paired* in the female

Y chromosome   The sex chromosome found only in the male

Suggested further reading

Bourne, G. (1975). *Pregnancy*. Pan Books, London.

Jolly, H. (1981). *Book of Child Care*. Sphere Books, London.

Jolly, H. (1983). *Common Sense about Babies and Children*. Unwin Paperbacks, London.

Kerr, M., Barron, M. and Tan, M. (1980). *Basic Baby Care*. Lloyd Luke Medical Books, London.

Kitzinger, S. (1982). *Birth over Thirty*. Sheldon Press, London.

Leach, P. (1983). *Babyhood*, 2nd edition. Penguin Books, Harmondsworth.

Llewellyn-Jones, D. (1982). *Everywoman. A Gynaecological Guide to Life*, 3rd edition. Faber and Faber, London.

Llewellyn-Jones, D. (1983). *Breast Feeding: How to Succeed. Questions and Answers for Mothers*. Faber and Faber, London.

Marshall, J. (1979). *Planning for a Family. An Atlas of Mucothermic Charts*, 2nd edition. Faber and Faber, London.

Nilsson, L., Furuhjelm, M., Ingelman-Sundberg, A. and Wirsen, C. (1977). *A Child is Born. Photographs of Life Before Birth: A Practical Guide for Expectant Mothers*. Faber and Faber, London.

You and Your Baby, Part 2. BMA Publications, London.

Your First Baby. Newbourne Publications in association with the Royal College of Midwives.

Index

Notes

Notes

Notes

Notes